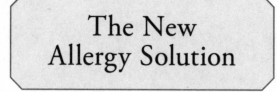

The New
Allergy Solution

The New Allergy Solution

■

Supercharge Resistance, Slash Medication, Stop Suffering

Clifford W. Bassett, M.D.

AVERY
an imprint of Penguin Random House
New York

AVERY

An imprint of Penguin Random House LLC
375 Hudson Street
New York, New York 10014

Copyright © 2017 by Clifford W. Bassett
Penguin supports copyright. Copyright fuels creativity, encourages diverse voices, promotes free speech, and creates a vibrant culture. Thank you for buying an authorized edition of this book and for complying with copyright laws by not reproducing, scanning, or distributing any part of it in any form without permission. You are supporting writers and allowing Penguin to continue to publish books for every reader.

Most Avery books are available at special quantity discounts for bulk purchase for sales promotions, premiums, fund-raising, and educational needs. Special books or book excerpts also can be created to fit specific needs. For details, write SpecialMarkets@penguinrandomhouse.com.

Library of Congress Cataloging-in-Publication Data

Names: Bassett, Clifford W., author.
Title: The new allergy solution : supercharge resistance, slash medication, stop suffering / Clifford W. Bassett, MD.
Description: New York : Avery, 2017. | Includes bibliographical references and index.
Identifiers: LCCN 2016058535 | ISBN 9781101980583 (hardcover) |
ISBN 9781101980606 (ebook)
Subjects: LCSH: Allergy—Alternative treatment—Popular works. | BISAC:
HEALTH & FITNESS / Allergies. | MEDICAL / Internal Medicine.
Classification: LCC RC588.A47 B37 2017 | DDC 616.97/3—dc23
LC record available at https://lccn.loc.gov/2016058535
p.   cm.

Printed in the United States of America
1 3 5 7 9 10 8 6 4 2

BOOK DESIGN BY TANYA MAIBORODA

Contents

■

Part 2 ▪ The Allergies

Part 3 ▪ New Ways

Foreword

∎

"This is going to be the worst allergy season in decades, perhaps ever!"

I can't tell you how often I've heard that story pitch in my three-plus decades as a medical correspondent for network television stations in New York and Philadelphia. Actually, I've heard that pretty much every single year. And the reasons for this purported allergy apocalypse are as varied as the weather: It's been a very dry winter/spring, it's been a very wet winter/spring, it's been unusually warm or cold or sunny or humid—you get the picture.

It's not that the public relations folks or allergists pitching those stories are dishonest or aren't well-meaning. It's that the rationale for the awful symptoms that allergy sufferers were experiencing was a moving target, crafted to fit the particular weather pattern that year. It's enough to make one a little cynical.

But what was always missing from those myopic explanations was something to help me convey to the general public *why* they were sneezing, rubbing their eyes, and going through a box of Kleenex a day—and, more important, what they could do to feel better. In other words, allergy sufferers—and that is the right word—need to *understand* their condition more fully and clearly, its causes and possible remedies, so that they can participate in their treatment. An educated patient is a far more willing patient, and ultimately a happier patient.

That's where *The New Allergy Solution* comes in. Here, for the first time, is a clear and concise description of allergies—the many types and causes, why you have them and your kids or spouse don't, what makes them worse and especially what works, and doesn't work, to get better.

Think of *The New Allergy Solution* as a kind of comprehensive owner's manual for your eyes, nose, throat, and sinuses—or at least for how pollen, food, medications, cosmetics, and other allergens affect them.

Over the years I've referred many people, including my own children, to Dr. Bassett. He looks at each one of them as a human being with a puzzle to be solved, because every person's allergies and solutions are going to be different. And solve them he does. Almost invariably, I also end up explaining some aspect of their allergy or treatment to them, not because Dr. Bassett didn't or wouldn't, but because they forgot to ask or didn't want to bother him. Now *The New Allergy Solution* does all that and more: It really answers all the questions anyone with allergies could ask, and a few they didn't think to ask.

Wow, what a relief! Not only will this book help countless allergy sufferers; it will save me tons of hours explaining allergies to friends, family and colleagues. So, on my behalf as well as that of all the sneezers and coughers out there, thank you, Dr. Bassett. You have done us all a great favor!

—Max Gomez, Ph.D.

New World

Chapter 1

Trigger Happy

■

What's Going On?

These days, spring springs earlier than it used to—*much* earlier: A study in the *International Journal of Climatology* (I'll assume you do not have a subscription) reports that, since the late 1940s, spring in the United States has been arriving earlier and earlier—summers, too—at a rate of more than 1½ days per decade. Which means that spring now starts approximately 10 days earlier than it did right after World War II. In Europe, the creep is similar. It's estimated that by century's end, early-onset spring will arrive more than three weeks earlier than it did just two to three generations ago, in some places nearly a month earlier; the effect on coasts tends to be more pronounced. With this change comes a longer growing season, which for allergy sufferers means lots more sneezing, wheezing, itching, and other annoying, frequently debilitating challenges. (Allergy tends not to get the "respect" that other medical conditions do; it's often portrayed as an inconvenience rather than a sometimes life-altering situation.) In my practice, I see many patients—young, older, middle-aged—who have never before had seasonal allergy but are experiencing it for the first time. The question so many of them ask me: "Why is this happening?" The answer is one of the main reasons I was driven to write this book.

We are in the midst of an allergy explosion. An estimated 30 percent of Americans, or roughly 100 million people, suffer from allergy and asthma; a Gallup study puts the figure at 50 percent. Globally, allergy affects 20 to 40 percent of the population. The rate in urban environments has increased for the past half century. In the United Kingdom, it's estimated that up to half of all kids suffer from some allergic condition. Once upon a time, you knew a few people with allergies, maybe more than that if your family or neighbors were genetically unlucky enough to have a disposition (more on the genetics of allergy in chapter 2). Now? Probably you know, or know of, five to ten times that number. While many are born wired for their allergic condition, it may be that the environments we now inhabit, both outdoor and in, the behaviors we engage in, the products we use, and the foods we consume have all changed enough in a short time that we are confronted by a genuinely new reality.

The uptick has occurred not just in one or two kinds of allergy. It spans the spectrum. It's seen in seasonal allergies and allergic respiratory disease, including asthma. Between 2001 and 2009, the number of Americans diagnosed with asthma grew by over 5 million, across all demographics. It's seen in food allergies. The CDC says that food allergy in children rose by half again, between 1997 and 2011. The rate of peanut allergy doubled in the last decade. The European Academy of Allergy and Clinical Immunology reported a 700 percent rise over the last decade in allergic reactions among European kids.

Why is this happening? In many cases, allergy "triggers"—the source of the scourge, exposure to which sets off an immune system reaction ranging from unpleasant to activity-limiting to debilitating to deadly—have gotten bigger, badder, and way more prevalent. Ragweed, the central culprit behind fall hay fever for those residing in regions with seasonal climates, is growing faster and bigger in many places, and blooming longer, with more pollen per plant and possibly more potent allergic potential. Combine this with other environmental troubles, such as human-generated air pollutants, and it creates a potential synergistic, amplified impact on your health.

Poison ivy today can be found more widely, and it's generally bigger and more potent, too. Even our mix of trees has altered the (allergy) landscape. In 1950, the native American elm, once the most popular "street tree" in neighborhoods across the United States and other countries, was a modest shedder of insect-transported pollen. But then Dutch elm disease ravaged the elm population, killing off billions—yes, billions—of these trees in the 1960s and '70s. Among their replacements were hardwood species like London plane sycamore and Norway maple, and a greater proportion of male trees, selected largely because they shed less, making it easier to keep streets, sidewalks, and yards clean—but they also produced more allergenic, wind-conveyed pollen. Says renowned horticulturist and author Tom Ogren, "In many areas today, tree pollen makes up more than 70 percent of the total urban pollen load."

Wasps, whose stings can cause allergic reaction ranging from swelling of the skin to hives to potentially deadly anaphylaxis, arrive earlier in the season and stay later. Fire ants, mostly a fixture in the South, seem over the past decade and a half to be moving gradually north and west. The mostly tropical triatoma, commonly called the kissing bug, is spreading northward. Mosquitoes are more prevalent in many areas, and their incubation time in certain regions has grown shorter. Of course, mosquitoes can cause harm far greater than allergic itching and swelling, such as West Nile virus, chikungunya,[1] dengue fever, and the confounding, often devastating Zika, the last three of which are on the rise. Forests are flourishing in the eastern United States—good news, right?—but that contributes to an increase in the deer population, thus an increase in deer ticks and cases of Lyme disease. In the last fifteen years, the number of annual Lyme cases in Canada has increased from roughly forty to seven hundred; two decades ago, ticks lived and reproduced in two areas in Canada, today in thirteen. The Lone Star tick,

---

1. While the incidence of chikungunya has risen in selected areas, including Asia, it has dropped in other places, particularly the U.S. and its territories, where interventional strategies have succeeded (http://www.who.int/mediacentre/factsheets/fs327/en/).

whose name bespeaks a southwestern habitat, is spreading north and east; its bite may trigger allergy to red meat, a particularly elusive condition to identify.

The reason behind much of what I've just chronicled is mostly climate change, or increases in "extreme weather." But climate change is hardly the only cause of the rise in allergy frequency, severity, and complexity. There are new threats in the air and water; in our food, homes, and offices; and on our bodies—our own "microenvironments"—that simply did not exist twenty or so years ago. These factors combine to make diagnosis more complicated. For example, people exposed to ozone plus ragweed allergen likely experience greater illness than those exposed to only one of the two—and it's less simple to get at the root, or roots, of what's going on. Our natural balance—by which I mean nature itself and our own individual nature—has been altered. When that happens, we may become overloaded, and an overreaction by the immune system becomes much more possible. A study by Quest Diagnostics shows that our rate of sensitization to common allergens—really, the first step in becoming allergic—has increased.

The range of increase in allergy is broad. So are the causes for the surge.

SIX BIG REASONS THAT ALLERGY IS RISING

A new weather map/seasonal calendar: We may be in the midst of an evolving "pollen tsunami." Climate change has led to higher temperatures, longer growing seasons, and increasing levels of greenhouse gases, meaning more carbon dioxide, meaning more pollen-loaded plants and flowers.

Globalization, particularly of food: Today, we can enjoy an endless menu of foods, imported from all over the world—and I'm not even including GMOs, or foods treated with pesticides or other pathogens to preserve freshness; I mean the incredibly wide array of fresh or well-preserved food. As consumers are exposed to a greater variety of culinary ingredients, there's a heightened chance we'll be affected by some of them. Global travel and trade are responsible for other burdens, such as the introduction of the mosquito-borne tropical disease chikungunya to Florida; and bringing, from Japan to the United States, the Asian tiger mosquito, a "vector" (agent) in the transmission of pathogens behind dengue, chikungunya, yellow fever, and Zika.

Changing habits/exposures/stresses: Allergy caused by nickel, among other metals, is suddenly a problem, though hardly a surprising one given our habit of being attached every waking hour to a cell phone or other metallic tech device. So many new substances are present, and present in new combinations and concentrations, and only a microscopic percentage have been evaluated for the effects they may cause when we're exposed to them. According to the Natural Resources Defense Council, more than eighty thousand chemicals currently in use in the United States have *not* been tested for their effect on human health—and that's just the individual chemical, not how they might interact in combination, or when used in ways different from what was intended. One example? Liquid flavorings in e-cigarettes are classified by the Food and Drug Administration as "Generally Recognized as Safe" (GRAS), but that's for oral consumption; the potential toxicity of these additives when inhaled has not been tested.

Overmedication: Many allergy medications that once required prescription are now sold over the counter. This may lead to overmedicating and an embrace of "symptom management" over diagnosis and treatment of root causes. Also, while the great majority of adverse reactions to drugs are not allergic in nature (they're mostly predicted side effects), up to 15 percent of reactions are, and virtually any drug may cause an allergic response.

Overcleaning, or the Hygiene Hypothesis: Our use of hand sanitizers and the like could be lowering resistance, particularly for the young.[2] A Bristol, England, study of fourteen thousand children showed correlation between frequency of hand-washing and likelihood for developing

---

2. As I completed writing this book, the US Food and Drug Administration announced a ban on certain antibacterial chemicals used in body and hand washes, and speculated that some of these ingredients may do more harm than good.

asthma. A German study found that children raised on farms had lower risk for allergy (though there can be multiple explanations for this); two new US studies show a similarly protective effect of the farm/rural lifestyle. Another study showed that kids raised for their first year around two or more dogs and/or cats were less allergically sensitized to such animals, and less sensitized generally later in childhood. A decrease in prevalence of childhood infections leads to increased prevalence of allergic disease. (The hygiene hypothesis is sometimes known as the biome depletion theory.) By overscrubbing the environment to which infants and toddlers are exposed, we may be weakening their immune systems. (The hygiene hypothesis does not appear to be behind the rise in asthma, and cannot be used to explain many health trends.)

Altered environments: The allergy increase is particularly noticeable in industrialized nations, especially cities. Tightly sealed, energy-efficient homes and offices often have less ventilation, with more dust and fumes from the carpets, furniture, and cleaning products trapped inside. The relentless march toward urbanization means greater exposure to pollutants from vehicular emission, a highly likely cause of respiratory disease. (A century ago, one in five people lived in urban areas; by 2030, that number is projected to be three in five.) An American Lung Association "State of the Air" report from 2012 to 2014 found that more than half of Americans, or 166 million people, inhabited the nation's 418 counties with unhealthful air pollution levels, a potential trigger of asthma attacks (and other unhealthy conditions). The majority of trees and shrubs now sold and planted in the United States are male, because homeowners often cut down trees that shed seeds (female) and leave standing those that don't (male), a tendency sometimes called botanical sexism. Over time, urban forests in the United States, Canada, and elsewhere have become much more allergenic (and more male-female imbalanced). And the growth of golf courses and gated communities full of lawns and flowers means that certain places—e.g., Arizona and Palm Springs—are no longer allergy-free havens.

These developments and more have ushered in an outright allergy surge.

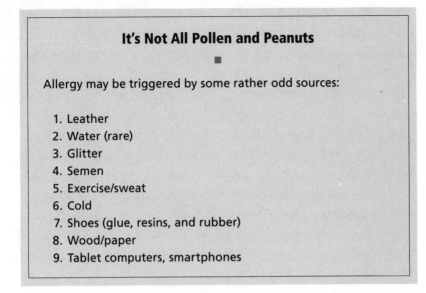

It's Not All Pollen and Peanuts

Allergy may be triggered by some rather odd sources:

1. Leather
2. Water (rare)
3. Glitter
4. Semen
5. Exercise/sweat
6. Cold
7. Shoes (glue, resins, and rubber)
8. Wood/paper
9. Tablet computers, smartphones

This list of six reasons does not include other possible modern-era causes for the increase in allergy, such as Western inflammation-boosting diets, the rise in obesity rate, occupational hazards, and more.

It's . . . Complicated

By many measures, then, allergy is more prevalent and damaging than when we were young and when our parents were young. Allergy is now responsible for more physical discomfort, lack of productivity, and overall life stress than it was years ago. In the United States, allergies are the number six cause of chronic illness. In a world inundated by new, often unregulated substances and products, and new ways of doing things, notions long viewed as unabashedly positive—eating adventurously, maintaining excellent personal hygiene, planting and enjoying flowers and trees—are being challenged for the dangers they might pose (though in many cases, they *can* improve one's health profile).

In short, things have grown more complicated. I experience it daily in my office. No longer do I see the case of the simple runny nose, the result of garden-variety hay fever that I treated so often when I started my practice more than twenty years ago. Instead, I, and my fellow allergists, tend to be confronted by more complex conditions, ones that are "multifactorial." As I tell patients, when working to understand and treat allergy today, one plus one rarely equals two. It could equal one hundred. By that, I mean the answer could be in your individual physiology, in the way the problem unfolds, in the treatment, in all of them. Allergy doesn't come with just primary symptoms (e.g., itching, redness, watery eyes) but also secondary symptoms (e.g., chronic sinus infection, nasal congestion, difficulty breathing). Certain substances or behaviors are not by themselves allergic triggers—alcohol, exercise, nonsteroidal anti-inflammatory drugs—yet if you're in their presence, they may increase the likelihood of an allergic reaction/anaphylaxis. I think of patients who react to allergens not through ingestion but mere contact or even inhalation—like Diana, whose extremely serious (and previously unknown) allergy to shellfish likely landed her in the hospital simply because she passed through an open kitchen where paella was being cooked. Similarly, my wife can get an outbreak of poison ivy merely by being in close proximity to it. I think of the three patients I've had in just the last six months who are allergic to beer—actually, an ingredient in beer (two are allergic to hops, one to malt). I think of the numerous patients I treat who have "comorbid" conditions—more than one chronic disease or condition, at least one of which may still be unrecognized, making the root cause of the suffering difficult to pin down. Many recent studies show that atopic dermatitis—eczema—is associated with food allergy. Another study, this one of children, showed an association between anemia and eczema, asthma, hay fever, or food allergy. Figuring out the often inscrutable immune system (which is at the heart of allergy and many other conditions) is made harder by the fact that you may have not only multiple symptoms but multiple triggers. Many people with asthma also have allergies; severe allergy is a significant factor in asthma development. *Allergy march* is the term we use to describe the progression from the earliest evidence of allergy to the development of other allergies and asthma: If you develop one allergy, there is a strong tendency to develop others. For example, eczema appears in about 10 percent of American children. Up to 80 percent of them will develop asthma or allergic rhinitis (the umbrella term for seasonal allergy and year-round sensitivity to dust, pet dander, mold, cockroaches, and more). Infants with food allergies are likelier than those without to develop asthma. The allergic march looks as if it's becoming a parade.

Obvious answers are growing less commonplace. Maybe the answer often prescribed in the past—medication—is necessary but not sufficient. Maybe the answer is (a) medication, plus (b), (c), (d), and (e), which represent avoidance, modifications to environment and behavior, and more.

Why Allergy Is Trending

The rise in allergy is not a phenomenon that has just reared its head. It's simply become more pronounced. In developed countries, the prevalence of allergic rhinitis began to creep up around the 1870s, continuing to rise for about eighty years. The asthma rate rose in the 1960s, and over the next three to four decades increased approximately tenfold. Part of that rise is due to improved awareness, diagnosis, and training by health care and urgent care providers, and in school and camp settings, too. And the rise is in some ways a mystery: After all, air quality in many places has improved, and crucially, the rate of smoking, thus the rate of secondhand smoke exposure, has broadly decreased.

Why these changes? Let's take a further step back for some historical perspective, and establish what got us here. Numerous developments in how and where we live—many of them quite spectacular for the overall health and well-being of the human species—have played vital roles in the rise of allergy. More than two hundred years ago, immunization was introduced to control infectious diseases, saving countless lives. The dawn of the twentieth century saw the separation of drinking water (meaning water used for cooking and washing, too) from sewage, and better treatment and control of food to prevent bacterial infection. Around 1920, we first enjoyed such leaps forward in hygiene as chlorination, a decline in hepatitis A infection, and eradication of most parasitic worms and malaria in Europe and the United States. Life gradually became better, then outright "easier." In 1935, we started furnishing our homes with more carpets and sofas, havens for allergens. The mid-1950s saw improved conditions for mite and mold growth, a stunning increase in the number of homes with television, and the accompanying increase in hours spent watching it, meaning more time spent indoors, less time out. The 1960s brought an array of antibiotics. As American family life changed, so did the American diet. The 1970s brought a rise in obesity. Everything from the decrease in average size of the family unit to greater reliance on antibiotics and overall reduction in our exposure to dirt, germs, and other potential pathogens may help to partly explain the rise in allergy.

Over the last two centuries, the developed world has enjoyed these profound changes; now it's the developing world's turn. There, allergic rhinitis and asthma began to shoot up about thirty years ago. Eczema has achieved much greater levels among children worldwide, perhaps as high as 20 percent.

Now, it would be madness to condemn outright what the Industrial Revolution, modern medicine, and their aftermath have done to society; we must acknowledge what they have done *for* society. The bulk of these developments—far more sanitary conditions, protection from difficult weather, individual choice, to name just a few—have led to resistance to some of history's most pernicious killers, such as cholera, tuberculosis, and strep throat, thereby reducing the incidence of certain lethal diseases, in many instances to close to zero. Our water has gotten generally cleaner (in most big cities, anyway). Collectively, we enjoy better health and longer life. We live in less pain and discomfort, in more ease. And even well-formed studies may nudge us at times to reach possibly unwarranted conclusions: For example, are farm children, who on average spend lots more time outdoors than most kids and are more exposed early on to certain germs and infections, less allergic because of that? Or because they're less exposed to urban scourges like cockroaches, mold, and diesel-choked air, which are associated with higher rates of allergy and asthma?

Still, as good as we have it now, even the most marvelous-seeming developments have downsides. There is no free lunch. In fact, it now turns out that that lunch may contain some food or additive that makes you or your child break out, for the first time ever. Or it's something in your home, or a medication you take for relief for something else. Triggers can be found all over. Two decades ago, I had one Manhattan office. Today, I have three, all busy, virtually all the time (though especially from April to June, prime allergy season on the East Coast); numerous colleagues have also never seen their practices this busy. Although my patient demographic is just one snapshot of the larger population, in the years since I began practicing, I now see more complex issues, from an increase in body piercings and tattoos, which can lead to allergic skin reactions, to exposure to an ever-increasing number of personal and skin care products and chemicals, which include new synthetic flavors and fragrances. These developments, coupled with the big changes mentioned previously, mean one thing:

This is not your parents' physical environment. We live in a new allergy landscape, with new allergy mysteries to solve and address. To do so, we could use a new allergy solution.

Taking Control

You worry about yourself, your children, other family and friends, and wonder how conventional allergy treatments, particularly medication, can deal with the damage wrought by this new world. For many people, the "old" approach to treatment may not suffice.

Why, then, are the millions suffering from allergies, asthma, food intolerance, and more, in this differently complex landscape and airscape, generally unaware that the thinking about and treatment of these conditions have changed significantly?

Good news: Our knowledge and approaches have improved. There are constructive new ways to manage allergy. If you've come to this book because you or a loved one suffers from allergy and/or asthma, there is great reason for optimism. There may be no "cure" for your allergy but in many cases it may be preventable. And I believe that nearly all cases of allergy are treatable. As I've seen in my practice time and time again, a program that includes improved diet, exercise, de-stressing, and overall health awareness (along with proper medication) correlates—if often only anecdotally—with less, and less severe, allergy.

It's perfectly natural to get confused or overwhelmed by what you're expected to know. Yet knowing more—and we do know much more than we did even just a decade ago—is a gift. Allergists, immunologists, general practitioners, and medical/scientific researchers are adjusting to meet the new allergy reality. If prevalence and complexity are spiking, then so, too—like some collective, ever-adjusting immune system—is our ability to respond. Thanks to continual advances in research, a greater and more accessible network of information, resourceful and thoughtful doctors, and the increasing benefits of Big Data analysis, our present-day allergy crisis has helped to spawn what I call a "new allergy solution," one that I have been using with considerable success on my patients. It's great that the average allergy sufferer now just has to turn on the TV or radio news, or tap her smartphone, and within seconds can find out the day's pollen count. It's great that, if need be, she's able to pop an over-the-counter oral antihistamine before she walks out the door.

But there's much more that we can do than just that.

We're recognizing new allergy patterns. We're developing new approaches and tools, such as immunotherapy. With new knowledge and an openness to multimodal tactics, we find that many conditions are conquerable, even quite simple.

The most important development of all is that you are thoroughly capable of understanding your condition, and should be invited to partner in making yourself better. My patients want more than just to sneeze less; they want to garden again, to partake in the activities they love and that make life enjoyable.

An example: In the United States, no food or ingredient in the last generation has been more demonized for its seemingly increasing capacity to cause allergic reaction, potentially to a life-threatening degree, than the peanut. (Gluten and lactose would probably round out some Axis of Food Intolerance/Allergy Evil.) Yet we now know that in many cases, perhaps most, peanut allergy may be preventable. A study led by George Du Toit compared more than five thousand Jewish children in the United Kingdom and the same number in Israel and discovered that the former were ten times more likely to be peanut-allergic. The two groups of kids were comparable in genetic background, social class, and exposure to other potential causes of allergy, like pollen and house dust. So what root difference between the cohorts likely caused the different outcome?

By nine months of age, the study found, approximately seven in ten Israeli infants were eating peanuts. (Peanut-rich Bamba is the most popular snack in Israel, purchased regularly by an estimated 90 percent of families there.) In the United Kingdom, the figure was one in ten. Could this finding help to explain the peanut allergy spike in the United States, United Kingdom, and Australia? One of the study's coauthors, Professor Gideon Lack, along with the Learning Early About Peanut (LEAP) team, followed with another study, published in 2015. It found that early introduction of peanut into the diet was associated with a very significant decrease in the development of peanut allergy in very young children who were at increased allergy risk.

I tell this story not merely to alert you to a promising piece of news but to point out a fact that I find nearly as intriguing: The first study was published in 2008, nearly a decade ago. Yet almost none of the mothers of very young children I see, and for whom this is a potentially important development, are aware of the study. Or the one from 2001 that may suggest a disparity in peanut allergy prevalence in the United States versus China, possibly explained by differences in the predominant method of cooking peanuts: In China, peanuts are mostly fried or boiled; here, we more often dry-roast them. ("Roasting uses higher temperatures that apparently increase the allergenic property," claims the Mount Sinai School of Medicine study.)

As you might expect, there is caution around the whole issue. The science isn't 100 percent. New data appear to support or sometimes refute universal recommendations concerning food allergy. Will the findings hold? In many circles, food avoidance in the first months of a child's life as a way to lower food allergy risk is seen as intuitive, conventional wisdom. But that view may be more nuanced, as new studies come out. And when health consumers are not aware of new, scientifically validated information, it can have a profound impact. That United Kingdom study of a decade ago, for example? Its significance extends well beyond the maligned peanut. In 2008, a report by the American Academy of Pediatrics found that there wasn't enough evidence for them to advise women with children at high risk for allergy (i.e., having at least one parent or sibling with allergy) to avoid potentially allergenic foods during pregnancy or lactation; such avoidance did not appear to lower their offspring's risk of developing allergic disease. A number of pediatric societies across Europe agreed with the findings. (Such dietary avoidance, it should be noted, may reduce eczema in the child's early life.) A very recent study suggests that food allergy risk to siblings of kids with food allergy is "only minimally higher" versus the general population. One of the most frequent questions I get is, "My child has food allergy—what's your recommendation for his little brother/sister?" My patients should know, as I learn it, how pertinent studies can impact them, even as we are careful with this new information.

Now, I don't expect the average citizen to comb allergy journals for cutting-edge knowledge and practices. That's our job. But there's a huge opportunity for physicians and allergists to significantly reduce the suffering of patients. As you will see, many proactive strategies remain inconclusive—don't show cause and effect—in part due to varying qualities in the research. And we're often slow to accept what seems increasingly clear. Even today, when the impact of nutrition on health is so much better appreciated, its inclusion in medical school curriculums, including many of the most elite, often remains a near-afterthought. Lots of promising medical research is unshared with the public or gets underreported, and the information is left to be discovered, somewhat scattershot, via the Internet and on TV health news segments.

That's why I wrote this book. The disconnect between the information that's usable *right now* versus what is often being advised and followed is unacceptable. My new allergy solution is simply this: *explaining, simplifying, demystifying, debunking,* and *integrating* all the exciting new information that's out there. It's amazing how much just doing that can help—though as you'll see, it's hardly "just doing that"!

If you're yearning for a solution that's a collection of radical ideas that are promising, potentially amazing, but yet to be adequately proven: It's not. It's about moving beyond merely neutralizing the bad. It's about promoting the good. It's about providing the best, most up-to-date information, including recent developments and findings, which will allow for an informed, productive conversation between you and your physician, allergist, obstetrician, child's pediatrician, and/or other medical specialists you rely on for current approaches regarding allergies. It's about confirming truths and dispelling myths.

My new allergy solution is about you wanting more options, so that increasingly you feel as if it's *your* treatment, rather than a protocol that's been forced on you without much consultation. Many of my patients, including lots of millennials, want treatments that fit their lives. They don't want to feel "sick" or even, if possible, to take traditional medication. Perhaps that's one reason why increasing attention has been given to allergy sublingual (under the tongue) immunotherapy (SLIT), or drops, which are allergenic extracts such as pollen, pet dander, molds, etc., to help build tolerance to the allergen and thus reduce allergic-type symptoms: It can be administered at home. The goal is not just to make things better but to make allergy care part of your normal routine, or at least as minimally disruptive as possible.

I am driven by the belief that wellness and a whole-body approach, rather than disease management or merely symptom management, are crucial. When you work out, you can't expect to be toned, strong, and pain-free unless your core is strong. Sure, you can work on your biceps or your calf muscles. But that will help only so much to improve your overall physique. The same is true, I believe, with allergy care. Your core inputs—exposures, stress level, sleep, diet—must be quality. Yes, you can suffer from allergies even if you are otherwise in fine shape. But for so many patients, improving that core improves their overall resistance and ability to heal.

I don't claim to be the inventor of any of the principles undergirding this approach, only that I have used and combined the best of these. While I've talked about topical allergy issues during appearances on the *Today* show, *Good Morning America*, NBC *Nightly News*, *The Dr. Oz Show*, NPR, Fox News, and more, I have long wanted to lay out my larger, comprehensive approach, and relate the experience of my own patients. This book is driven by science that is relatively straightforward, tested, credible, and applicable. Where there are ideas that are exciting but as yet thoroughly proven, I'll say so. My patients want to know more, to be involved in and take greater control of their health generally, and do it in a way that's cost-effective and long-term. (Not everyone is willing: I occasionally encounter an asthmatic who will bravely make dietary and other lifestyle changes—but won't stop smoking. I have to tell her that her improvement probably won't be significant.)

The first time I see a patient, I often find it useful to establish a baseline of her allergy knowledge. How much does she know about the conditions, environments, behaviors, etc., that typically cause reactions in allergy sufferers? What does she know about ways to improve the situation, particularly non-medicinally? My role is to be a medical detective but also a medical educator. The more you know about common triggers and next steps, the happier you'll be, the more control you'll enjoy, and the better able you'll be to dispense wisdom to your loved ones.

In most cases, I find, my patients don't at first know what they ought to.

How much do you know about allergy? Take this simple quiz. (If you don't score well, don't worry—that's why you're here.)

WHAT'S YOUR ALLERGY IQ? (ANSWERS ON PAGE 24.)

1. Which steps best help to reduce seasonal allergy exposure and symptoms?

   _____ a. wear waterproof shoes

   _____ b. wear a hat

   _____ c. line-dry your clothes

   _____ d. b and c

2. What are the best plants and flowers to have if you have seasonal allergies?

   _____ a. azalea

   _____ b. begonia

   _____ c. bulbs (tulip, iris, poppy, and daffodil)

   _____ d. orchid

   _____ e. all of the above

3. What is the culprit that hits many seasonal (spring) allergy sufferers *first* (in places with seasons)?

   _____ a. tree

   _____ b. ragweed

   _____ c. weed

   _____ d. mold spores

4. Which climate condition is most associated with higher levels of seasonal pollen?

   _____ a. rain

   _____ b. dry air

   _____ c. clouds

   _____ d. wind

5. Which has the greatest effect on worsening seasonal allergies?

   _____ a. fresh fruits and vegetables

   _____ b. wheat

   _____ c. flaxseed

   _____ d. buckwheat

6. The best way to clean the air in your home is by
   _____ a. running a window fan
   _____ b. using a cool-air humidifier
   _____ c. turning on the air conditioner and/or HEPA air filter
   _____ d. regularly sweeping and dusting surfaces

7. When is best to work in your garden if you have seasonal allergies?
   _____ a. early morning
   _____ b. mid-afternoon
   _____ c. early evening
   _____ d. after it rains

8. Which factor most likely affects your allergies?
   _____ a. air temperature
   _____ b. humidity
   _____ c. ozone
   _____ d. breezy and windy days

9. What is the best way to reduce the load of seasonal allergens entering your home on a high-pollen day?
   _____ a. create a "pet-free" bedroom
   _____ b. brush/wipe your pet before entering the home
   _____ c. pretreat with your allergy medications before exposure
   _____ d. all of the above

10. Which symptom usually helps to tell the difference between allergy and a cold?
    _____ a. stuffy nose
    _____ b. cough
    _____ c. headache
    _____ d. itchiness

11. The number one estimated food allergy among adult women is
    _____ a. cow's milk
    _____ b. egg
    _____ c. shellfish
    _____ d. tree nuts

12. If you use anti-allergy medications, it is ideal to take them
    _____ a. before allergy season begins
    _____ b. after your symptoms develop
    _____ c. year-round

13. Which is a possible cause of sneezing?
    _____ a. pollen and/or mold spores
    _____ b. spicy foods
    _____ c. bright sunlight
    _____ d. all of the above

14. Acupuncture may help to reduce allergy symptoms.
    _____ a. true
    _____ b. false

15. Moving to a new geographical area, particularly the Southwest, will likely reduce many triggers for allergy and asthma.
    _____ a. true
    _____ b. false

16. Eating local honey helps relieve symptoms of seasonal allergy.
    _____ a. true
    _____ b. false

17. _____ is a great natural mosquito repellent.
    ____ a. oil of lemon eucalyptus
    ____ b. canola oil
    ____ c. avocado oil
    ____ d. olive oil

18. As a pet owner with mild to middling allergy, you can reliably improve your condition by getting a certified hypoallergenic cat or dog.
    ____ a. true
    ____ b. false

19. As we age, we tend to get
    ____ a. more allergic
    ____ b. less allergic

Know More

What's the likeliest solution? Medication, probably. That's often needed in the short-term, and perhaps long-term. But the new allergy solution comprises numerous strategies I have searched out and developed over the last two decades, an integrative approach that includes avoidance, dietary changes, exercise, homeostatic practices, and changes in environment, indoor and out. In my practice, I bring visuals, stories, and information. I won't just advocate using an immediately available medication; instead, I might say, "Let's do an anxiety questionnaire. Let's see what might be at the root." I have seen my patients navigate remarkable turnarounds, not just in dealing with short-term problems (e.g., "allergy face" features—visible changes due to allergy—to be discussed later, in chapter 4), but in their long-term health and well-being.

In today's global world, it's crucial to know what's going on in different cultures, for the clues and insights they may provide. If the prevalence of peanut allergy in China is significantly less than it is in the

United States, shouldn't we know what they're doing in China? Let's use everything at our disposal.

This book covers most major allergies, and some minor ones, too. It covers allergic asthma and asthma-related conditions. I will tell stories of patients I've treated and explain how they were able to progress from the suffering condition that brought them to my office, to the better, healthier place they ended up. In telling these stories, I believe that you can gain real knowledge to help yourself and others lead more comfortable lives.

Part 2 of this book is divided by allergy type. In each chapter, I will share the most beneficial information and thinking. I'm sure I'll share some things that you already know. I believe I'll also alert you to information that's new and helpful. Some information is necessarily repeated, either in different chapters or within sections in chapters. Choices were made about where to discuss certain subjects—for example, poison ivy is discussed in detail in chapter 7 (Skin Allergies) rather than chapter 5 (Outdoors and Seasonal Allergies). Discussion of asthma and allergic asthma, and about children and early life, can be found throughout the book, where relevant.

Part 3 is devoted to a broader discussion of health changes that, both generally and specifically, can help you live a healthier, more energetic, happier life. Which of the newer protocols enjoys a scientifically, medically significant level of evidence about their benefits? Which look to be well on their way? Which may be of little to no help? We'll sort through the landscape.

It's imperative to understand that so much of what we're learning about allergy, as with so much in medicine, is in flux—that is, with new research studies being conducted and published all the time, we're confirming things we weren't sure of, or overturning conventional wisdom, starting to see things in a new light. Five years from now? We will know more than we do now.

Before we jump into fixes and treatment, it would help for you to understand the root problem. How does allergy work? What defines it? First, let's know the enemy.

ANSWERS TO QUIZ:

1. b. wear a hat
2. e. all of the above
3. a. tree
4. d. wind
5. a. fresh fruits and vegetables
6. c. turning on the air conditioner and/or HEPA air filter
7. d. after it rains
8. d. breezy and windy days
9. c. pretreat with your allergy medications before exposure
10. d. itchiness
11. c. shellfish
12. a. before allergy season begins
13. d. all of the above
14. a. true
15. b. false
16. b. false
17. a. oil of lemon eucalyptus
18. b. false
19. b. less allergic

As this book went to press, revised national guidelines were released to address the possible "prevention" of peanut allergy. These guidelines, based on the most up-to-date research, discuss new recommendations on early introduction of peanut in infants. Before making any changes to your child's diet, including peanuts, it is imperative to consult and work closely with your pediatrician and/or allergist.

Chapter 2

Defining the Terms, Diagnosing the Problem

■

How Allergy Works

You come in contact with a particular substance—an allergen, usually a protein—to which you and a small subset of the population have, or will eventually have, a reaction. Your immune system thinks this substance presents a threat, so it devises a defense, at least for the future, by manufacturing an antibody called Immunoglobulin E, or IgE. The IgE attaches, or binds, to mast cells, found in most tissues of the body, such as near blood vessels and in the mucosa (lining) of the skin, respiratory tract, gastrointestinal tract, and other areas. Without knowing it, you are becoming allergically sensitized to the offending substance.

Newly prepared, your body lies in wait for the next interaction with this allergen, this supposed enemy. I sometimes liken allergic sensitivity to a gun with its trigger cocked: The gun won't go off until the trigger is pulled. When the interaction happens, the allergic reaction is set off—the allergen attaches to the IgE antibodies on the mast cells, which "degranulate," meaning they are triggered to release an inflammatory substance called histamine and other chemicals, and these set off throughout your body to fight the enemy. Body tissue is affected; blood

> ## More Boys Than Girls, Until It Isn't
>
> ◼
>
> About 70 percent of allergic individuals experience their first reaction before they turn twenty years old. Boys are far more prone than are girls; in the preteen years, it's about twice as prevalent in boys. Gender disparity narrows until the rate evens out by age thirty.

vessels and the mucous membranes expand. Symptoms manifest in areas where histamine was released—dry skin, red and watery eyes, itchy throat, runny nose, etc. Generally, symptoms emerge within seconds or minutes of exposure, to hours. Some studies estimate that up to 20 percent of the time there's a second wave of symptoms. This reaction, which typically erupts within twelve hours after the initial attack subsides, can still be quite severe, possibly (though rarely) fatal.

It's Fascinating, and Confusing

Interestingly, you can become sensitized to an allergen without experiencing symptoms. In other words, a blood test would register an above-average level of IgE antibody to a particular allergen—yet there's no external sign of its presence; no symptoms. In such a case, you are considered allergically sensitized: You are at increased risk of developing allergic symptoms in the future but have not yet exhibited them. What does that mean in real terms? That only *some* allergically sensitive individuals—not all—will develop symptoms.

Somewhat relatedly, two different conditions may present with symptoms similar enough to confuse us. An allergic reaction may be misdiagnosed to be non-allergic, or vice versa. The common cold and a sinus infection, for example, are often mistaken for allergy, and the reverse mistake also happens. The confusion is even more likely during pollen season.

ALLERGY OR COLD/SINUS INFECTION?
THE 4 W'S AND TELLTALE SYMPTOMS

Pattern	Cold/Sinus Infection	Allergy
WHAT (Onset and duration)	Cold and/or infection symptoms develop within a few days, onset is abrupt, may last up to 7–14 days	Gradual or immediate onset, depending on exposure and level of one's sensitivity to allergen, so symptoms may resolve or persist after exposure.
WHEN	Anytime of year, but more common during late fall through late winter	Anytime of year (e.g., seasonal, indoor triggers), though the appearance of some symptoms may last months.
WHO	Children and adults	Children and adults
WHY	Viruses (hundreds of varieties)	Seasonal pollen, indoor allergens and irritants
SYMPTOMS		
Nasal congestion or stuffiness	Frequent	Frequent
Body aches and pains	Not uncommon (especially with the flu)	Never
Fatigue	Common	Sometimes, especially if sleep is impaired due to severe nasal congestion
Fever	Not uncommon	Never
Watery, itchy eyes	Rare	Often
Painful throat and discomfort swallowing	Often	Occasional
Cough	Common	Sometimes

Misdiagnoses happen all the time. If day after day you wake up tired during allergy season but don't make the connection, perhaps you think it's some low-level virus. But maybe it's blocked nasal and sinus passages, which cause sleep-disordered breathing, which means you're not getting enough REM sleep, which affects brain processing and productivity, which affects quality of life. When it's a child experiencing this, it impacts cognitive performance, which impacts performance more broadly, including in the classroom—and before you know it, parents, teachers, and administrators are scrambling down paths presuming entirely unconnected explanations. I'm not suggesting that kids diagnosed with ADHD are actually just experiencing chronic allergy. One study reported that boys with ADHD are more commonly seen to have allergies and asthma than those without. Of the many kids and teens I see who have ADHD, those with poorly controlled allergic rhinitis have an extra hurdle during the school day: Their bothersome allergy includes symptoms like nasal obstruction, which means they can't breathe optimally, particularly at night, which means daytime inattentiveness, lack of alertness, and drowsiness. Indeed, for those of any age, living with allergy, especially when it's not well controlled, can result in poor sleep, potentially creating an inattentive or foggy state that resembles ADHD-type behavior patterns.

I'm fascinated by how we arrive at conclusions that turn out to be inadequate or incorrect because we didn't gather all the facts. *Allergy masquerader* is the term for something that *looks* like allergy but is in fact something else. Recently, an eighth grader spent a day with her classmates in Central Park and came away suffering itchy, watery, red eyes. Her mother went to the local pharmacy to get antihistamines and topical eye drops, thinking the red eyes were caused by pollen. Alas, the girl got no relief; after a trip to the ophthalmologist, it turned out to be an infection (which resolved after a few days of antibiotic eye drops). As a young allergist-in-training, I saw a patient with a rash that looked like hives, and I was quietly confident that after doing an examination and running some diagnostic tests, I would know exactly the allergy causing it . . . only I was wrong. The causes of the rash were strep throat and tonsillitis, not an uncommon diagnosis. It's possible for some conditions to be misdiagnosed as more serious than an allergy, leading to overtreatment. Or maybe there *is* an allergic trigger—but we initially chose the wrong one. Someone may get hives and be certain it's caused by her new skin care product, when it's actually triggered by something unexpected like sunlight, vibration, alcohol, cold temperature, and/or exercise (more on those in chapter 7).

To understand allergy, one needs to understand the immune system, which is at the core of many health conditions and diseases. (It might be quicker to list what the immune system *doesn't* impact than what it does.) During my medical training, when I had to settle on a concentration, it wasn't hard: immunology. Inflammation, viruses, enzyme deficiencies, cancer, asthma, autoimmune disease, arthritis, some types of diabetes—the immune system is at the center of so much of it. Yet because of its scope, there is still so much we don't know. It's often a mystery. The "dual-allergen exposure hypothesis" is just one instance of a fascinating riddle: Some children—kids with eczema, for example, who have disrupted skin barriers that may allow proteins from potential allergens to penetrate—may be exposed through the skin to food allergens, such as peanut oil (likelier to occur with the cold-pressed variety), and develop allergy. Yet kids who *eat* these foods when they're very young may develop a tolerance for them. Which will win—allergy or tolerance? And why?

Sometimes, we're stumped. Of the patients who come into my office, one-third have already been to another doctor or clinic and, for one reason or another, have received insufficient relief from their suffering.

In some instances, the term *allergy* is misused by patients and even doctors as an umbrella term for other conditions. In some instances, terms such as *intolerance* and *sensitivity* are used instead of *allergy*. There are cases where they are clinically different from allergy, and some where they are not. I will make the distinction, where helpful.

Why the Overreaction? Evolution

You have a basic grasp of the "how" of allergy. What about the "why"? Why is this whole bodily debacle set off by something as "harmless" as pollen?

One possibility is that, molecularly, certain otherwise harmless proteins in food or in the environment, such as pollen, are similar to certain more obvious nemeses, such as parasitic worms. Our bodies evolved to fight against and protect us from these harmful parasitic worms (among other much bigger multicellular invaders), but these parasites no longer exist in our environment the way they did. (We have not rid ourselves of parasitic worms, and probably won't—they've been around for millions of years; they pose more of a health threat in the developing world.) Still, our immune system is wired for a fight—for *that* fight. Those who subscribe to the hygiene hypothesis believe that oversanitized environments expose the young to a much narrower range of microbes than is needed by the infant, still-developing immune system; it is partly through contact with a variety of microorganisms and bacteria that the individual learns how to respond appropriately when confronted by these substances. In a sense, this early exposure teaches the immune system when and how to fight. In the absence of this early "germ training," when an individual encounters something harmless but similar to a true nemesis, the system hyperdefends. A person who goes into anaphylactic shock from ingesting a peanut may be an example of the immune system grossly overreacting, to a possibly fatal degree, to a nonharmful intruder. It's bodily friendly fire. Dr. Nicholas Furnham of the London School of Hygiene and Tropical Medicine, the leader of a study exploring this phenomenon, reasons that "allergy is the price we pay for having immunity to parasites."

Pollen is not a saber-toothed tiger. It is not even pinworm, which causes itching but is not particularly hard to get rid of. Dr. Graham Rook noticed that after pinworm was eliminated nationwide as a health threat in the United Kingdom, allergy spiked. He surmised that as we

---

Have More Kids, Sneeze Less

■

One study found that those in smaller families are likelier to get hay fever than those in larger families.

---

eliminate intestinal parasites and mycobacteria, we also mess with the balance of a harmony that monitors cells (called T cell regulators) that train our immune system not to react, or overreact, to each and every pathogen it encounters, or else a different type of cell (called T cell effectors) will start doing their antagonistic thing. The scientists behind the study refer to their theory as the Old Friends Hypothesis (a refinement of the hygiene hypothesis), which suggests that by losing our "old friends"—these microorganisms—we have made ourselves, in some ways, more vulnerable.

For significant subsets of the population, the discomfort and pain caused by allergy may be an unfortunate, cranky by-product of evolution dealing with mostly defunct invaders. If certain parasitic worms and protozoa are no longer part of *today's* Enemies List (at least in the developed world), what is? It's useful for allergists like myself, for general physicians, and for you, the health consumer, to know which common substances out there have the greatest potential for triggering our bodies in harmful ways.

The Hygiene Hypothesis: A Fine Theory but Is It a True Theory?

Not everyone agrees with the premise, or at least the real-world impact, of the hygiene hypothesis. For one, profound changes in hygiene in northern European cities predate evidence of an increase in kids' asthma rates (though these changes seem to correlate with the incidence of hay fever). For another, asthma has risen in certain African cities whose level of hygiene lags that of major cities in the United States and Europe a century ago.

Others support its premise. In one study, dishwashing by hand correlated with lowered risk for developing asthma, eczema, and nasal and eye allergies at seven to eight years of age; the same correlation wasn't there for machine dishwashing. There's the study that showed that kids who grew up on farms had a decreased risk of allergy, and stronger lungs as adults. (As one person has said, "It's the 'farm' effect, stupid.") Further studies are looking at this hypothesis, and we may soon have a higher degree of confidence that it's true.

I am a strong believer in the hygiene hypothesis. But what can you do about it? We live in the world we live in, oversanitized as it is. Whatever "improvements" we might make to counter that scrubbed environment may have minimal effect, since so much of the benefit to the immune system accrues in the first months of life. How does a concerned parent of a newborn, or a prospective parent, approach this situation?

If you're inclined to accept the premise of the hygiene hypothesis, then here are four findings to consider (though please read the "disclaimer" that follows the list):

1. Two or more pets at home, early in a child's life, may lower the risk of pet allergy, as well as asthma, eczema, and rhinitis. (It's not clear if it's more associated with dogs than cats.)
2. It's possible that avoiding day care, for fear that your child's exposure will lead to her catching something, could do more bad (allergically speaking, of course) than good.
3. The exclusive use of water that's boiled/sterilized, for fear of germs, may reduce the chance of (some) very young children to build robust, healthy immune systems.
4. Antibiotic overuse in a child's first year can raise the risk of asthma and some allergic conditions, perhaps even doubling it.

If you follow these steps, will allergy play a smaller, even nonexistent, role in your life? As a doctor, I can't say that. After all, point #1 is not a fact—yet an array of studies seems to support the notion. Point #2 comes with a caveat: Exposure to certain pathogens, like strep, is associated with serious disease. Point #3, also: There are risks to unsterilized water—e.g., exposure to certain contagious viruses and bacterial infections.

Still, it's worthwhile, maybe even life-changing, for you to know what's happening in allergy research. This way, you—employing a very healthy dose of common sense, and in active dialogue with your health care provider, your child's pediatrician, or another medical specialist—can make choices that may lead to meaningful differences.

COMMON ALLERGIC TRIGGERS AND IRRITANTS

Indoor Triggers

1. dust mites
2. mold spores
3. cat dander
4. dog dander
5. feather or down
6. cockroach
7. mice
8. outdoor pollen brought indoors
9. strong fragrant scents—potpourri, cleaning products, room fragrance, scented candles, etc.

Outdoor Triggers

1. tree pollen
2. grass pollen
3. ragweed/weed pollen
4. mold spores
5. air pollutants

Skin Triggers

1. fragrance
2. preservatives in skin care cosmetics and products
3. formaldehyde and releasers
4. acrylates (nail products)
5. metals (nickel, gold, etc.)
6. antibacterial compounds
7. dyes (PPD)
8. sunscreen
9. glues
10. tanning agents
11. shampoo
12. detergents
13. disinfectants
14. rubber
15. cement
16. poison ivy or "rhus dermatitis"
17. clothing or textiles
18. leather
19. steroids (topical skin creams and/or ointments)

Food Triggers

1. peanut
2. tree nuts
3. egg
4. milk
5. shellfish
6. fin fish
7. soy
8. wheat
9. seeds (e.g., sesame)

Drug/Medication Triggers

1. antibiotics—sulfonamide, penicillin, amoxicillin, ampicillin, quinolones, cephalosporins, others
2. narcotic pain medications
3. non-steroidal anti-inflammatory drugs (NSAIDs)—ibuprofen (Advil, Motrin, etc.), naproxen (Aleve, Anaprox, etc.), others
4. aspirin
5. muscle relaxants given intravenously—succinylcholine (Anectine), vecuronium (Norcuron), and other anesthetic agents (Tracrium)
6. blood pressure medications
7. ACE inhibitors
8. antiseizure medications—carbamazepine (Carbatrol, Epitol, Tegretol), lamotrigine (Lamictal), phenytoin (Dilantin, Di-Phen, Phenytek), others
9. chemotherapy
10. HIV drugs—nevirapine (Viramune), abacavir (Ziagen), others
11. monoclonal antibody therapy—cetuximab (Erbitux), rituximab (Rituxan), others
12. radio-contrast agents, commonly used in diagnostic radiology studies, or X-rays

Stinging Insects, Bites

1. honeybee
2. yellow jacket
3. wasp
4. hornet
5. fire ant
6. triatoma ("kissing bug")
7. mosquito (can cause Skeeter's syndrome)

Sinus and Respiratory Infection

1. viral
2. bacterial
3. fungal

> ## On Vaccines
>
> ■
>
> If you believe, as I largely do, in the truth of the hygiene hypothesis, it does not necessarily follow that you are anti-vaccination. Vaccines help to protect our own children and all children, and greatly reduce the potential spread of infectious diseases.

Why Am I Afflicted and You're Not?

What's the best advice you can give someone (so goes the joke) to prevent their suffering from allergy? Choose parents who don't have allergy.

There's obviously a broad range in the severity of allergic condition. But the difference between those with and without often comes down, simply, to genetics.

Some "guesstimates" say that if neither of your parents is/was allergic, you have an estimated 10 percent chance of being allergic. If one parent has/had allergy, your likelihood rises to 25+ percent. If both parents are/were allergic, the likelihood rises to 50 to 60+ percent. If both parents have the same allergic condition, the risk rises to as high as 80 percent.

Yet while genetics plays a predominant role, we recognize, like never before, that environment may play a significant role, too, in the development and exacerbation of allergy—hence, in many ways, this book.

So when a patient appears in my office having experienced one or more reactions (respiratory, skin, etc.), I start with some basic knowledge. I know that the underlying condition is the result of genetics, environment, or both. Often I make an "allergy family tree," which diagrams the genetic part of the equation, helping to confirm a link or refute it. It's like ancestry.com for allergies (and asthma), only much simpler. While the allergy tree is not conclusive, it can be usefully suggestive. For example, if you had an asthmatic relative, are you likely to

---

Work Hazard

■

Two of my patients suffered the same condition: "contact allergy," which causes blisters and eczema. I realized that they were both buyers in the fashion world. Was it occupational? Yes: They touched lots of fabrics, and because of the many dyes used in today's textiles, they each developed the allergy. For both, I recommended that they wear cotton or silk gloves—fashionable ones, of course.

---

be one, too? If your mother, father, and grandfather had asthma, and you come in wheezing, you have a strong allergy and asthma disease predisposition. If your allergy tree shows no asthma among siblings, parents, or grandparents (except in rare instances, it's not necessary to retreat further than two generations), and you live with your father, a smoker, and there are cats in the house, and you come in wheezing, the cause is likely environmental.

The question, then, is, which part(s) of the environment? Cigarette smoke may be the entire cause of your problem. Or the cats may be the entire cause. Or maybe both cigarettes and cats contribute. Or maybe strong dust control measures are needed, too. Or it's unseen mold.

If there's no strong genetic component, personal history may still hold important clues. In many ways, that's where my work really begins.

Identifying Through History: Questions and Tests

One reason allergy care appeals to me is the "solving mysteries" part. I have enjoyed that since I solved my first medical mystery: I was the subject, age nineteen. As a sophomore at the University of Maryland, I was on spring break in Fort Lauderdale, Florida, when one night I found myself coughing and breathing so badly that I ended up in the emergency room. Although a dose of epinephrine got me back to normal, I was stumped at how I had gotten there, and why I ended up right back there the following night. Searching through the available details, I remained stumped—until my cousin, who was hosting me, told me that she had (very kindly) cleared the cat litter box from the guest room where I was sleeping. I deduced that I had an obvious, severe, and previously undetected cat allergy. I had no visual evidence of the trigger, but my body sure noticed.

In solving my own medical mystery, I understood the value in paying attention to external stimuli, hidden clues, and personal history. (Soon after, I learned that my father, unbeknownst to me, had also suffered from severe cat allergy.) Over the remainder of my undergraduate and medical school years and beyond, my enthusiasm for figuring things out would blossom into a commitment to discover better ways for patients to deal with severe, often unexplained physical discomfort and life-threatening medical situations. And I wanted to find solutions that might make more sense than the by-the-book, short-term fixes that so many doctors prescribe.

Today, my team and I combine (a) observations we make, (b) answers to questions we ask, (c) information we already have, and (d) results from tests we can administer, all to get a much fuller picture.

(a) *Observations we make*—like the quality and level of severity/discomfort, size (body-wide versus localized) and location of rashes, hives, redness, swelling, and eczema, and the extent of itchiness.

(b) *Answers to basic questions*—like:
- How often are you symptomatic?
- How long do your symptoms last?
- If you have a rash, is there itching, too?
- How is your sleep?
- Is it impaired enough to affect normal daily activities?
- What foods make up your diet?
- What products and accessories regularly come in contact with your skin?

- What chemicals might be present in your home or office environment?
- What is your history with antibiotics? What medications are you using?
- Have you had lots of ear, sinus, or respiratory infections?
- . . . and more.

(c) *Information we already know*—like:
- Skin allergy to a product usually manifests as rash, hives, breakouts, and itchiness.
- Allergic reactions to medications and foods are usually rash, swelling of the tissues, hives, potentially threatening breathing trouble, and shock.
- The pattern of a rash on the skin, hands, face, and eyelids signals dermatitis or something else.
- Seasonal pollen, molds, and indoor allergens target organs: eyes, nose, sinuses, and the lungs.
- . . . and more.

(d) *Results from tests we can administer*—like:
- Patch test
- Skin prick test (SPT; intradermal test)
- Challenge test (food or drug)
- Blood test (formerly called RASTs, for radioallergosorbent tests, when radioactivity was used)

I find this part of my job—information-gathering, which leads to informed diagnosis—the most satisfying. Detective skills honed over decades enable me to determine the true triggers of an allergic condition, after which we devise a team approach that emphasizes patient involvement, for an optimal solution and plan of action.

Collaboration with You, the Team, Other Doctors

Recently, I found myself in the hospital for chest pain, the source of which remained unclear for days. At first, the doctors took an EKG and surmised it was a heart attack. (I told them it wasn't.) Then a specialist was called in. Then another. And another. In all, *twelve* specialists weighed in. It appeared that there was little, if any, communication between or among them. Eight scans were taken, five or six other tests administered. After all that, they figured out what it was—a simple virus.

Aside from the experience making me even more empathetic to what patients go through, I could not believe how little sharing went on between the doctors—yet why was I surprised? They're specialists! They're magnificently trained to see through their own important, but narrow, lens. Yet today, there's a huge opportunity for general practitioners, specialists, and allergists, to work together when needed to help in individual cases, and also to help the general public. The reason many doctors don't share this information with patients has to do with a flawed system. If you're a patient on a managed care health plan, as many Americans are, then it's simply not possible for a general practitioner to sit with you, chat, get a personal history, and work at demystifying your problem when a dozen patients are sitting in the waiting room.

When a cancer patient is first absorbing what's going on, she is often advised to bring an advocate to consultations, because that companion might be better equipped, mentally and emotionally, to take in what is being said. We do this for more serious diseases. Why not for ones like allergy, though, that deeply affect the quality of day-to-day life, and whose source is often shrouded in mystery? Sharon, a patient experiencing congestion and itchiness, came for a couple of office visits over the course of one month, yet the source of her problem had eluded our efforts so far. On her third visit she brought her sister, who within two minutes of sitting down pointed out that Sharon had not long before changed to using a feather pillow, a fact that Sharon had overlooked, and we discovered that allergy to feather and dust mites was the culprit. Each patient's profile is different. That's why I try to know what's going on with each of them. Leading up to a patient's initial visit, it can be helpful if she records details around her symptoms so that we have more to go on.

The allergy solution I follow is anything but a "siloed" approach. We look at the whole immune system, and the crucial issue of inflammation. How do weather, the environment, nutrition, etc., affect those with allergic conditions? Are some of these factors co-conspirators in causing or exacerbating the original condition? What immune system irregularities or hypersensitivities can we uncover?

The more detailed a picture you have of your likely condition, the more ready you'll be to make modifications that can lead to optimal relief, greater health, and well-being.

Chapter 3

What Does Prevention Look Like?

■

More Than Just Chemicals

Toward the end of my undergraduate career, I took a psychology course—how the mind works and how it potentially affects the body. That's when I embraced the idea, obvious today, that if we doctors interact positively with patients, if we communicate clearly and show real empathy, the patient's healing arsenal may actually expand. To be the sort of allergist I wanted meant I had to be good primarily at three things: gathering evidence, connecting dots, and acting kindly toward my patients. From the start of my medical career I knew that the only way to answer key questions about my patients' discomfort was by accumulating facts, and the best person to help with that was the patient, the one actually suffering. We are detectives together. When a patient reviews her diet with me, I literally copy down each ingredient as I prepare an evaluation of potential triggers.

That college psychology course, and my reading and thinking beyond it, influenced how I saw the body. At a recent seminar, an expert spoke about how many cases of hives may be stress-induced, and how a significant percentage of individuals with hives experience rampant anxiety. Doesn't it make sense to treat the deeper potential source of a skin problem that, to the outside world, looks like "merely" an allergy? Of course it does. Stress, after all, can trigger an asthma attack. One needs the short-term medication fix, just as I desperately needed medication for my breathing issues in Florida. But to really get you on a healthier, happier track, we need to dig further, so we can figure out the best ways to boost your immune system and resistance and, where possible, reduce medication.

Your approach has to be multimodal because people live complex lives, and there may be multiple sources to your suffering. Every system is connected—nervous, respiratory, endocrine, the gut—not to mention how the mind and mood may affect physical outcomes. The root cause may lie in your physical/biochemical makeup; in your personal environment; in the larger environment; in a combination of these—like the recent study from the University of British Columbia that suggested that children whose mothers when pregnant with them were exposed to significant air pollution are at greater risk of developing asthma by age six. My interest in the multifactorial nature of allergy and the multimodal nature of treatment inspired me to coauthor a paper on the effect of mood and mental state on asthma.

My new allergy solution is based on an appreciation of the big picture, something we're fully capable of seeing but that our medical system is generally not set up to address in an efficient way. Once we dig and get at the nature of the problem, we arrive at the ultimate, and most rewarding, part of my job: prescribing a course of action that relieves discomfort and pain, and creates the opportunity for a healthier, better life.

Diagnosis is really just the first step, the end of the beginning. Once we believe we may have solved the mystery, we proceed to the reason you've come: relief.

What now?

Prevention? Cure?

In traditional allergy care, we want to provide relief of symptoms, as well as to significantly reduce the risk of recurrence; if allergy does recur, we want to reduce its severity and frequency. To do these, we follow four principles for "managing" allergy:

1. *Avoidance of trigger factors*—e.g., don't eat foods known to cause reactions, don't venture where poison ivy is rampant, enlist someone who's *not* allergic to rake leaves and mow your lawn.

2. *Environmental/behavioral modification*—e.g., remove damp carpet from the basement; wear big sunglasses outdoors; open windows, use air-conditioning or employ other means for improved ventilation of indoor space.

3. *Pharmacotherapy*—e.g., use medication to relieve symptoms; help asthmatic breathing with nebulizer/inhaler; employ newer therapies, such as biologics, in cases of severe asthma and chronic hives.

4. *Immunotherapy*—e.g., provide injections, tablets, or drops to treat allergen-specific issues.

The holy grail is prevention. The prevention of the development of an allergic disease altogether is what we aspire to, more than "just" maintenance. It may seem impossible; in a sense, we'd be trying to outsmart our bodies. Yet for all that today's ever-changing environment may bombard us with—new foods, new chemicals and drug interactions, air and water of a changed composition—we seem poised, eventually, to truly shrink particular allergic diseases from the landscape. Can allergy be prevented? Not yet, but perhaps a hopeful, qualified yes for the not-too-distant future. "Qualified" because for certain patients, conditions, and stages of life, prevention is not possible (anyway, we have yet to figure it out), and the immune system can be maddeningly inscrutable. "Hopeful" because the more we learn, the more we see how modifications within our control may curtail development of many of our respiratory, food, drug, and skin allergies.

We're hesitant to use the word *cure* when referring to allergy. "Cure" is misleading, and often implies the problem will never return, which simply can't be guaranteed. If you have a predisposition to allergy, maybe one type goes away forever—but you may develop other allergies. Cure implies that the patient no longer bears any risk of disease but, as we know from illnesses like cancer, even eradicating all signs and symptoms within the body does not guarantee the disease won't return. We might try a protocol on a patient and their condition goes away for years. Take the widespread use of the vaccine to prevent chicken pox. It succeeds in significantly reducing the likelihood that you will suffer the effects of the chicken pox or Varicella virus. However, nearly one-third of all Americans will go on, at some point in their lives, to develop shingles (aka herpes zoster); each year in the United States there are roughly one million new cases. If you recovered once from chicken pox, you can get shingles—and the risk increases with age. As you age, then, I can't accurately say you're cured of chicken pox because, simply, it sometimes reappears in a different form. Recent guidelines report that allergies to certain foods, such as milk, egg, wheat, and soy, are more likely to resolve during childhood than others, such as peanut, nut, fish and shellfish, which often persist through adulthood. We're not exactly sure why—but neither can we say that we did anything to cure it because we didn't. With food allergies in children and adults, the only successful strategy in your control is avoidance. I strive to educate my patients in which culprits to stay away from and how to reduce the chance of accidental exposure (much more on that in part 2).

There are other allergies, though, where the strategy goes beyond mere avoidance. The study I referenced earlier, which showed that children in Israel enjoy lower rates of peanut allergy than do children residing in the UK (who are otherwise similar in genetic background, social class and exposure to other allergens), and an important National Institutes of Health–funded LEAP (Learning Early About Peanut) study, which found that eating peanut early in life was associated with significant, persistent reduction in peanut allergic reactions, even after the very young children stopped consuming peanuts. Whether such observations can lead to preempting that allergic condition or others, thus a lifetime relatively free of one or more allergies that would otherwise have been present, is still not completely known. In such cases, we *still* can't use the word "cure." Maybe I'll say my patient's symptoms have resolved. It's not purely a semantic difference. It's an acknowledgment that unpredictable things happen.

Three Types of Prevention: Primary, Secondary, Tertiary

It's important to clarify the three types of prevention. (These can apply to a wide range of medical conditions, not just allergy and asthma.)

Primary prevention looks to stop the disease from even occurring. It's ground-level prevention—reducing and removing risks (i.e., exposure, behaviors), while enhancing resistance and promoting health so onset can't happen. It means altering the immediate environment and/or your relation to it. It aims to block sensitization by the immune system, thus preventing the development of IgE antibodies specific to that allergen. This level of prevention involves intervening before any evidence or appearance of the condition. Some examples are vaccines (e.g., for flu); smoking cessation, particularly during pregnancy and early childhood years; remediating homes to eliminate mold issues, and reducing indoor air pollution; and reducing/eliminating exposure to occupational-related irritants. Primary prevention may include one-on-one counseling, such as weight and nutritional counseling to help reduce obesity, which may benefit asthma control; and public health and awareness campaigns.

Primary prevention programs can reduce the overall cost—to you and the larger community—of treating a condition, should it occur.

Primary prevention may be characterized as proactive, not merely reactive. For example, what you do early in your child's life (e.g., not shielding her from certain bacteria; getting her to eat certain foods; breastfeeding, if possible, through the first four months; etc.) may make her more allergy-resistant in the future.

Secondary prevention looks to reduce the impact of a disease that is already present. It is about slowing or stopping disease progression through early detection, prompt treatment, and responsible follow-up. It's about encouraging you to adopt behaviors that limit the severity and frequency of recurrence, and pursuing strategies that return you to better health. Sensitization has happened; you have produced allergy antibodies. Allergic reaction may or may not yet have happened. The key question is: How can we keep this allergy from degrading your quality of life? A good deal of what might happen in the first two years of an allergic-sensitive baby/toddler's life could be considered secondary prevention, such as medical screening procedures that detect any early changes in a condition, thereby enabling us to reduce the likelihood that it develops. Other examples include: asthma screening (using breathing capacity tests), asthma questionnaires, and reducing exposure to indoor allergens (a measure that overlaps with primary prevention). One of the most exciting instances of secondary prevention is allergen immunotherapy, a treatment that helps build tolerance to a particular allergen, thus lowering your sensitivity to it and reducing symptoms over time.

Tertiary prevention looks to reduce the impact of the long-lasting effects of an existing condition. How can we help people to manage their health problems so they have maximum functionality and quality of life? The disease has already expressed itself acutely; now we want to modify risk factors to reduce the possibility of future complications. It's really more modification than prevention, aiming to diminish future bouts of symptoms (their frequency, severity, and duration). Some examples are altering your environment at home or work to reduce allergy triggers (e.g., creating a gluten- or food allergen–free kitchen); supplementing the diet of cow's milk–allergic infants and young children with hypoallergenic formula; using bed covers and mattress/pillow casings to lessen exposure to house dust mites and pet dander; reducing exposure to outdoor allergens (for those with allergies and allergic asthma); and medication for reducing inflammation.

We need medication to manage symptoms. We will need medical breakthroughs so that more of our approach is primary and secondary prevention, so that more of what we do is preemptive, not reactive.

If you feel that the disctinction between and among the three levels of prevention is fluid, even confusing: You are correct. For example, the flu vaccine may be considered both primary preventive strategy, as stated earlier, and also tertiary, since the vaccine is designed to prevent and/or reduce the most severe flu symptoms. One-on-one counseling may be considered primary, secondary, *and* tertiary prevention, depending on how far—or if—the condition in question has developed. The immune system is endlessly complex, even downright mysterious. There is debate about how much secondary and tertiary measures truly help. Some options even seem contradictory. For example, your sinusitis symptoms may be reduced by ridding yourself of indoor plants . . . but a well-known NASA study has identified houseplants that scrub indoor air clean.

Many of the avoidance strategies documented in this book may work very well, yet we don't have enough conclusive testing in many areas to say with complete confidence that some of the new techniques work, or work on a large enough segment of those who suffer from this allergy or that.

To simplify these complicated, even murky, terms, I'd say this:

- Primary prevention is to stop disease from starting.
- Secondary prevention is to stop disease from progressing.
- Tertiary prevention is to stop disease progression from worsening.

The chapters that follow deal mostly with the second and third types of prevention, but also a few primary prevention recommendations.

Short-Term, Long-Term

Some fixes, particularly medication, provide short-term relief; others, such as environmental modification and immunotherapy, provide longer-term relief. Patients often come back to my office on a regular, if infrequent, basis because they realize the benefit of *continuity of care*, as we refine our approach. For example, for many patients with hay fever, I recommend that they "pretreat"—start medication before the season starts. Why wait until tree pollen is airborne and allergy symptoms have appeared? It takes a few days for the medicine to kick in. This strategy enables the medication to stymie the release of histamine and other chemicals, significantly reducing the severity of symptoms, and possibly eliminating them for the season altogether.

In many cases, however, an approach becomes gradually less effective. When that happens, we want to revisit the issue and have a good plan B ready.

Any meaningful approach to good health—and I don't mean just for fighting allergy now, but for the overall health of body, mind, and spirit—necessarily combines short-term and long-term strategies.

Trends in Disease Treatment

Medical research will continue to uncover new facts and expand on strategies for fighting allergic disease, and that's great. For example, allergen immunotherapy has been a tool at our disposal for decades. Now, though, clinical trials have confirmed its effectiveness with allergic rhinitis, asthma, and venom allergy, and even more ambitious forms of immunotherapy are being evaluated.

More than just marching forward in our scientific/medical understanding, we also benefit from new patient-focused ideas about disease management, medication, and wellness that help to drive how health care professionals and patients pursue and embrace solutions. For example, there is little doubt that people increasingly see themselves as "health/wellness consumers," which is a very positive development. People want more choice. There is more demand for organic food and transparency in labeling (ingredients, GMOs, calorie counts, local farms, and how food gets prepared, etc.). There is interest in the benefits that healthful food can provide—whether it's plant-based diets, low-inflammation diets, or power foods that boost performance. There is more sharing of information, increasingly through social media, which provides guidance for those open to it. There is an appreciation for the gut-body connection and the mind-body connection. There is an eagerness for exercise as a de-stresser. There is an appreciation for what medicine can do—and what it can't.

It all goes back to that first "trend" I mentioned: The willingness to seek out information and use it. To be educated. To lead, or at least be an informed partner, in what you put into your body, and how you are willing to change your behaviors or modify your environment.[1] If you have allergic disease, you may want or need to go to an allergist or your own physician—or it may be unnecessary.

Part 2 of this book deals with diagnosis, causes, symptoms, symptom management, and other treatment for the range of common (and some uncommon) allergies and allergy-like conditions.

Part 3 addresses what's ahead in allergy treatment, from the likely to the speculative, and may take on relevant ways to promote overall health.

In the end, our goal is to minimize the effects of allergy as much as possible so that you can lead as full and energetic a life as possible.

---

1. Women patients, it's been my experience, are much more open to early intervention, doing what needs doing to their bodies or the household environment. Men are typically worse about addressing allergy and asthma symptoms, trying to tough them out, which often results in their using more medication.

Part

2

The Allergies

Chapter 4

Nose and Sinuses, Face, Lungs, Eyes: Some Basic Allergies

Allergy affects how you feel and look. I want to help you to feel and look better.

Among the most common, energy-depleting, life-diminishing allergies are those that impact the nose/sinuses, the eyes and the face; a lot of those also affect the skin—but that warrants its own chapter (chapter 7). These allergies are often not as debilitating as some—e.g., a severe peanut allergy—but still, if you're experiencing it, your outlook on the world can change, negatively, very fast.

Because of the interplay between and among these organs, symptoms manifest in numerous ways. One of the most frequent, frustrating conditions I see in my practice is what we call "allergy face," often seen in children: swollen, red eyes; puffiness and discoloration beneath the lower eyelids; rhinorrhea (runny nose); and mouth breathing. Allergy face is not exclusive to one allergy. It can affect you if you have rhinitis—but what kind of rhinitis? Allergic or non-allergic? Aspects that accompany allergy face—for example, sneezing and fatigue—are also common in sinusitis. Other symptoms, such as nasal and sinus congestion or diminished sense of smell or taste, are more common when you have nasal polyps.

So not all allergy-like symptoms are the result of allergy. There's allergic rhinitis (better known as seasonal or indoor allergy) as well as non-allergic rhinitis.

Making our assessment more complicated still, allergic rhinitis, to keep to this one example, which is inflammation of the lining of the nose, is often more than just a solitary condition, and may be associated with other conditions such as asthma, allergic conjunctivitis (allergy of the eye and eyelid), eczema, and Eustachian tube dysfunction.

That's why diagnosis is so important: We want to be as confident as possible that the treatment options we choose are truly addressing the root cause.

Is That a Solution—or Another Problem?

Dina, a twenty-five-year-old magazine editor, came to my office for an evaluation during the height of pollen season, complaining of increasing nasal and sinus discomfort, and presenting with swelling and bluish lines beneath her eyelids—an "allergic shiner" whose appearance is likely caused by blood pooling beneath the skin below the eyes from congestion. I couldn't see all that at first, though, because Dina wore cosmetic concealer to cover up the puffiness, darkness, and creases.

In doing so, she had made things worse: Some of the puffiness was *due* to the concealer. Testing revealed an allergic reaction to it. We also identified allergies to pet dander and house dust mites—indoor allergens, though it was outdoor allergy season.

I recommended that Dina modify her home: Make her bedroom pet-free, add a HEPA air purifier, and use a variety of short-term allergy and sinus medications, including a nasal steroid spray.

The unsightly puffiness and shiners mostly resolved within two weeks.

This chapter explores the triggers of some of the most common types of allergy that I, and my colleagues, see in daily practice. It also provides the path to short-term relief and long-term management and, ideally, reduction in incidence and severity. What does maximum, fast-working relief for allergy-related nose, sinus, and eye issues entail?

The Nose and Sinuses (Upper Respiratory System)

We tend not to appreciate the many vital functions being performed by the normal, healthy nose and sinuses, and what each does every moment. The nose filters outside air before it enters our lungs, keeping out invasive particles. It moistens the air, to around 75 to 80 percent humidity, to keep the airways from getting too dry. It heats up the air in the nasal cavities to approximately 98.6°F (37°C) so that the air reaches the lungs nicely warm. And the nose does this, in the average adult, by processing more than fourteen thousand liters of air daily. Overall, the nose plays an important part in our immune defense system. And of course it helps us to smell and taste.

When nasal allergy hits, important parts of this efficient system get messed up. The membranes of the nose and sinuses swell, resulting in symptoms such as congestion, sneezing, itching, postnasal discharge, and runny nose. Given the interrelated nature of the nose/sinuses and eyes, nasal allergy may also cause other maddening symptoms, including facial pain and red, itchy, watery eyes.

Put another way, when the nasal passages are confronted with an allergen, a "double whammy" occurs: The first response typically causes familiar nasal symptoms (runny nose, sneezing, and itchiness), which generally kick in quickly. Then—often—delayed and/or persistent symptoms occur, including nasal congestion and stuffiness, which interfere with optimal breathing, leading to nighttime sleep impairment. Many of those who suffer from nasal allergy, especially when it's not well-controlled, report sleep-related problems; a disorder such as sleep

---

Who's Got the Bigger Nose—Men or Women?

▪

Boy noses and girl noses are, relative to body size, about equally big. Then the male nose inches ahead during the teen years and by adulthood, relative to body size, it's 10 percent larger than the female nose. The reason? The greater amount of lean muscle mass that men possess. Building and maintaining that tissue demands more oxygen; a larger nose brings in more oxygen.

---

apnea may be associated with nasal allergy, prolonging the exhausting, debilitating punch of seasonal and indoor allergies.

We aim to recommend medications designed to reduce and/or prevent the array of allergy-triggered nasal and eye symptoms.

The Allergic Face and Nasal Allergy

What does an allergic nose *look* like? It's not always possible to know if you have allergies just by appearance. However, certain features are consistent with nasal allergy, and a doctor looking inside your nose—to see, for example, changes in the color of the tissues lining it—may identify them.

The most immediate giveaway is the "nasal salute." You repeatedly horizontally rub the nose's midsection until a crease is visible on the bridge of the nose. There may be clear nasal discharge; if infection is present, the discharge may be colored and generally thicker.

"Allergic shiners" are often another sign of allergy—and, yes, they look very much as if you've been in a fight. The lower eyelids are puffy and irritated, the result of nasal congestion: The veins normally drain from around the eyes, and when the sinuses get backed up, the veins dilate, swelling the surrounding tissue and darkening the skin just beneath the eyes. When you lie down, gravity can increase that fluid collection, deepening the shadowy look.

Another telltale sign are Dennie-Morgan lines, wrinkles that look like creases under the folds of the lower eyelids.

Other signs of nasal allergy include "long face syndrome" (adenoidal swelling from tissue that did not atrophy or shrink when the patient was a child, making for a droopy, tired look); nasal obstruction and postnasal drip, leading to persistent throat clearing; and nasal swelling that reduces airflow, leading to diminished sense of smell and mouth breathing.

That's a lot for me to go on—but I'm a determined detective, so I like to gather all my information before making a diagnosis of, say, allergic rhinitis. I'll ask the patient questions, such as:

Stop That Medicine

■

When Kenny came to see me years ago, I diagnosed him with mild pollen allergy and prescribed medication. He did not return and I assumed things had worked out. A couple of years later, Kenny showed up again, distressed. "Dr. Bassett, I saw you years ago," he told me, "and I'm still suffering. I don't sleep well. I'm always tired. My nose is so stuffed I wake up every night. I have the cold that never ends." After inquiry and testing, I discovered that Kenny was using—overusing, actually—a nasal decongestant spray. Instead of relieving his congestion, it made it worse, which contributed to his interrupted sleep and snoring. Because his breathing at night had become serious enough to wake him, he now had to deal with all the problems that come from bad sleep.

I told him to immediately stop using the spray. We switched him to an effective spray containing an antihistamine, as well as a steroid-containing nasal spray that eventually cleared up the congestion, allowing him finally to sleep through the night.

When did symptoms start? How long did they last? How have they progressed? Do they occur seasonally or year-round? Are there associated symptoms in the eye or pharynx (the cavity behind the nose and mouth)? Have there been repeated instances of sinus or ear infection? Are there asthma or chest symptoms? And maybe the biggest question of all: What do *you* think is the trigger?

I will also ask about the patient's family history of allergy; any previous allergy testing; use of medication, both prescription and nonprescription; any history of facial and/or nasal trauma; and any incidence of nasal/sinus surgery.

Non-Allergic Rhinitis

It looks like allergy . . . but testing does not pinpoint any specific seasonal or indoor allergens to classify this condition as allergic. Non-allergic rhinitis is a diagnosis made largely by exclusion; given your symptoms of nasal congestion, a runny nose or postnasal drip, I investigate various explanations (e.g., deviated nasal septum, structural problems, nasal polyps, infection, etc.). Other tests may be done (e.g., allergy skin test, blood test, CT scan of the sinuses). If the findings from all that reveal nothing conclusive, then non-allergic rhinitis is what we're left with. (Although the true cause of non-allergic rhinitis is unclear, it's thought to be associated with dilated blood vessels that line the nose.) In some cases, rhinitis may be both allergic (i.e., affected by triggers such as pollen, mold, dust mites, and pet dander) and non-allergic (affected by air pollution, dust, smoke, fumes, perfume and fragrances, alcohol, abrupt changes in temperature, etc.).

We want to arrive at the correct diagnosis quickly or we can't treat the condition effectively. For example, an allergy pill won't treat a sinus infection. Same goes for sinus meds for allergy. Conditions such as pregnancy, having low thyroid function, use of certain medications, deviated nasal septum, sinusitis, collapsed nasal valve, and nasal polyps may all cause nasal and sinus congestion, whether or not you have allergies.

The Mayo Clinic reports that one cause of non-allergic rhinitis is overuse of topical nasal decongestant spray (e.g., oxymetazoline); this condition is called rhinitis medicamentosa. In as little as three days of using these short-acting sprays (as my patient Kenny did), you may feel "rebound nasal congestion," which feels worse than the condition you were trying to fix!

Before you use decongestant spray, ask your doctor: How effective is it? How likely and adverse are the potential side effects? Which is preferable, nasal or oral?

OTHER CAUSES OF NON-ALLERGIC RHINITIS:

- infection—viral, bacterial, or fungal
- medication—aspirin, ibuprofen, beta- and alpha-blocker blood pressure drugs, erectile dysfunction meds
- hormonal changes—pregnancy, menstruation, hormonal contraceptives, thyroid disorders
- food (hot/spicy)
- alcohol
- cold (e.g., skier's nose)
- atrophy
- work irritants
- pollution smoke
- strong odors

Unlike the triggers for allergic rhinitis (hay fever), the ones just listed are not seasonal, thus symptoms may be felt year-round.

Treatment for non-allergic rhinitis depends on how much it bothers you. Mild symptoms can often be modified with a variety of low-key, home-type remedies. These include saline nasal sprays or gels, either prepared or commercially packaged to provide a cleansing, soothing, and/or moisturizing treatment to dry nasal passages, and to remove and/or thin out accumulated mucus.

Some of my rhinitis patients (non-allergic and allergic both) have genuinely benefited from nasal irrigation, along with other therapies, when allergies and/or colds or sinus conditions are present. The key is to use distilled, sterilized, or previously boiled water.

1. Put 1 cup water and ½ teaspoon noniodized salt into a small saucepan; cover it.
2. Boil for 15 minutes.
3. Cool to room temperature.
4. Pour solution into a glass jar or bottle.

Some individuals prefer using a nasal saline device, such as a neti pot. (It's important that the container start out perfectly clean—not just the solution.)

Angle your head slightly over the sink and gently introduce the device/bottle into the nostril. Some prefer to do this in the shower.

Nasal irrigations have proven popular, and may help to

- improve breathing
- improve sinus drainage
- reduce mucus and secretions, which may reduce source of future infection

There are potential disadvantages to nasal saline rinses/irrigations:

- The excessive irrigation may leave salt remains in nose.
- Nasal dryness may lead to nosebleeds.
- It takes work to properly clean and disinfect the device.

Consult with your health provider or specialist about when to do nasal irrigation, for how long, and the preferred device. Some solutions can be regular salt water, while others should be "hypertonic" for greater effectiveness—specifically, for when you have an infection during a cold, and need maximum mucus-eliminating power. The National Center for Complementary and Integrative Health reports "reasonably good evidence that nasal irrigation with saline can be useful for relief of seasonal allergy symptoms."

Some recent reports indicate that neti pot use may increase sinus infections, when used daily and for a prolonged period. One theory: In depleting mucus, you also deplete its infection-fighting potential.

Other steps for treating non-allergic rhinitis include OTC and prescription nasal steroids and antihistamines. A prescription antihistamine nasal spray may be even more helpful. OTC oral antihistamines relieve symptoms such as sneezing, itching, and runny nose but not nasal congestion. Read the label for instructions or speak with your health care provider if you are taking other medications. Your doctor may prescribe an "antidrip" nasal spray prescription, or ipratropium bromide, which often works on a drippy nose. Mild side effects may include dryness or irritation.

Available OTC nasal and oral decongestants provide relief in reducing congestion but may produce side effects that develop within days of use (as mentioned earlier). Oral decongestants typically produce more significant adverse effects, and in general should not be used, particularly if you have high blood pressure, cardiac disease, glaucoma, or urological conditions like prostate enlargement.

Are there complementary or alternative medical (CAM) approaches? Scientific evidence remains rather limited. Small studies have indicated that capsaicin, a compound found in chili peppers, may provide relief for nasal congestion, in non-allergic and allergic types of rhinitis.

Some symptoms in non-allergic rhinitis may signal a more urgent condition—e.g., acute infection—that requires evaluation and treatment. These symptoms include nasal bleeding, sudden blockage of one or both sides of the nose, thickened/colored nasal mucus associated with facial pain, headache, malaise, fever, and/or dizziness.

Longer-term complications may arise from non-allergic rhinitis, including nasal polyps, sinus infection, middle ear infection, diminished productivity, and daytime fatigue.

Allergic Rhinitis

This version of rhinitis, called hay fever or, in a tribute to its universality, simply "allergies," is triggered by known allergens, which cause the nose to swell and become inflamed, leading to symptoms such as nasal congestion, stuffiness and sneezing, and itchy eyes and throat. Allergic rhinitis may be of the seasonal/outdoor variety, where pollen and outdoor mold are the most obvious culprit triggers, or the year-round/indoor variety, where house dust mites, pet dander, indoor mold, and other home/workplace allergens are the likely causes.

Allergic rhinitis is thought to affect 10 to 40 percent of children and adults.

A favored treatment option for those with moderate to severe seasonal allergy: intranasal steroids, which curb inflammation and reduce nasal swelling. If your allergy is year-round? A nasal steroid may be used for longer periods, and I recommend that you be examined on a regular basis. At times I advise patients to start a course of medicines at least a week before experts forecast the start of pollen season; it may take a few days before the drugs really kick in. By medicating before the season's first contact with allergens, histamine and other inflammatory chemicals may remain unreleased, rendering symptoms less severe.

Nasal steroids are found in liquid form, like Nasonex, Nasacort AQ, Rhinocort AQ, and Flonase, and in dry/powder form, like Q-Nasl and Zetonna.

Some patients prefer liquid to powder; both types work.

Nasal steroids can also be used to treat non-allergic rhinitis and nasal polyps, reducing inflammation and swelling. As with all medication, nasal steroids come with possible side effects: dryness, a sensation of burning/stinging, nasal irritation. If you experience these symptoms, ask your doctor to prescribe another medication. Some patients do not like the taste. If you have conditions such as elevated intraocular pressure, nasal steroids should be not be used without consulting an ophthalmologist.

NASAL AND EYE ALLERGY MEDICATIONS

What They Do for You, and How

- *Oral antihistamine* reduces runny nose, sneezing, watery eyes, and itchiness of the eyes and nose. It provides relief for most people, though it's less effective for nasal congestion. Long-acting antihistamines are taken once or twice daily.

- *Nasal antihistamine* reduces runny nose, stuffiness, sneezing, and itchiness in both allergic and non-allergic rhinitis. Onset is quick, often thirty minutes or sooner, and may last up to twenty-four hours.

- *Nasal steroid spray* very effectively reduces runny nose, stuffiness or congestion, sneezing, and itchiness. It's usually sprayed once daily. Onset may take up to twelve hours. Duration may extend beyond twenty-four hours.

- *Nasal and oral decongestant* (only by prescription) reduces swelling of the nasal lining, reducing congestion. The onset for nasal spray decongestant is quick, within minutes (it's being absorbed through the nose, after all); oral decongestant typically starts to work within the first hour. The effect of both can last for hours. Potential side effects (with oral decongestants, and particularly in older adults or those with heart disease) may include heart palpitations, insomnia, and dryness of nasal membranes (from overuse).

- *Non-steroidal spray (cromolyn)* is generally less effective than nasal steroid spray. It's taken three to four times daily. If taken before exposure, it can prevent allergic symptoms.

- *Oral leukotriene receptor blocker (montelukast)* (only by prescription) is approved for the treatment of allergic rhinitis and helps to reduce sneezing, nasal congestion, runny nose, and itchiness of the nose. Generally, it's not as effective as nasal steroid spray. Onset is not immediate; it may take one or more days to deliver maximum benefit, and is taken once daily. Follow your doctor's instructions when this is prescribed for asthma and/or exercise-induced bronchospasm.

- *Ocular antihistamine (drops)* offers a reduction in symptoms including itchiness, tearing and eye redness due to allergies (some have anti-inflammatory, or mast-cell-blocking, effects). Onset is usually within the first hour and lasts up to twenty-four hours.
- *Ocular decongestant (drops)* reduces eye redness. Onset is fast and lasts up to twelve hours. Use for more than three days may be associated with irritation, dryness, and "rebound redness" of the eyes.

Sinusitis (Sinus Infection)

A number of sources point to a marked increase worldwide in sinus disease, including infections. Adults are likelier to get sinus infections, which can be acute or chronic. As always, it's important first to confirm what you have. Is it allergy? A cold? A sinus infection?

One sign of sinusitis is red, inflamed, swollen nasal mucosa (membrane). If nasal discharge presents thickened secretions and mucus of a changing color, that may suggest bacterial infection; antibiotics and other medication plus saline/salt water irrigation or nasal moisturizers may be called for. Other symptoms of sinusitis include nasal congestion, headache, facial pain, toothache (felt more by children), fever, and loss of taste or smell (which returns shortly). To examine the nasal and sinus cavities more extensively, we'll do a nasal endoscopy; if more severe or persistent symptoms exist, your provider may recommend an ear, nose, and throat (ENT) specialist, and/or order a sinus X-ray or CT scan of the sinuses.

If sinus discomfort is the result of the common cold, medication may be pointless.

If a sinus infection lasts briefly, it's acute sinusitis. If it lasts for twelve weeks or more, it's chronic sinusitis (or chronic rhinosinusitis). Prolonged infection may indicate nasal polyps, deviated septum, weak immune response—or just a stubborn infection that your body is having trouble clearing.

Positive steps to take when you have sinusitis:

- Drink fluids.
- Apply moist heat to your face (as directed by your practitioner or ENT specialist) multiple times a day (five to ten minutes each, using a damp, hot towel or gel pack).
- Take a steamy shower or hot bath so you can breathe in moist, warm air.
- Use nasal irrigation (either commercially available OTC or prepared at home as instructed).
- When blowing your nose, do so gently.
- Elevate the head of your bed to facilitate improved sinus drainage.
- If your room is dry, use a humidifier (if you don't have allergic sensitivity to mold and dust mites).

See your doctor about what course of treatment seems wisest—saline nasal irrigation, nasal corticosteroids, or antibiotics (when necessary). When seasonal or year-round allergens are the persistent trigger, as with allergic rhinitis, or when multiple medications are required regularly but produce little improvement, then the recommended course may be allergen immunotherapy—either injections, tablets, or drops for effective long-term improvement. If that doesn't help, then surgical intervention may be recommended. Complement these more elaborate approaches with prevention-oriented, environment-modifying techniques.

How can you reduce the risk of getting this condition in the first place?

- Wash your hands. Especially during cold/flu season, use alcohol-based hand-sanitizing gels.
- Stop smoking. Studies show that sinuses are irritated by cigarette smoke.
- Nasal irrigation with a neti pot and nasal or salt water solution.

Quick, Affordable Options

- Nasal ointments and gels may reduce nasal dryness.
- External nasal strips applied to the bottom third of the nose can alleviate congestion.
- Regular use of a neti pot plus steam inhalation may reduce some symptoms, which may reduce your need for antibiotics.

- Avoid pollen at peak times (if you have allergic sensitivity).
- Be careful when swimming underwater or high diving: These activities alter sinus pressure, potentially opening the way for infection.

Polyps

Polyps are small growths that may form in mucous membranes that line the nose and sinuses, and often indicate chronic sinus disease. Unlike polyps that grow in the bladder or colon, these are rarely cancerous. Particularly when small, polyps may cause no symptoms. Many patients have asymptomatic polyps: These are associated only with nasal blockage, not with recurrent or chronic infection.

Polyps may cause distressing symptoms such as the loss or decrease of sense of smell (which occurs in up to two-thirds of those with polyps) or taste, and sinus congestion, which can lead to poor drainage and infection. Other common symptoms include sneezing, postnasal drip, and altered shape of the nose. Polyps are twice as common in men, and risk increases as one reaches age forty. A child under ten with polyps should be tested for cystic fibrosis.

Nasal polyps can also be associated with chronic sinusitis, sensitivity to aspirin, sleep apnea, wheezing and certain types of asthma, and infection.

The cause of polyps is not entirely known. Some of us may have a genetic predisposition to developing them. Some researchers feel the connection with nasal allergy hasn't yet been made persuasively.

To confirm or rule out various possibilities about polyps and their root cause, ENT specialists or allergists rely on nasal endoscopy, imaging studies of the sinuses, and allergy tests and blood tests. Our goal is to reduce the size of the polyps or, ideally, eliminate them—though they often recur. They are treatable by medication such as nasal corticosteroids, oral and injectable corticosteroids, and other medications. Surgery may be an option.

How can you possibly control symptoms or polyp growth?

- Manage your allergies and asthma.
- Avoid extreme irritation to the nose (especially in work/industrial settings, where fumes and smoke may be present).
- Enhance nasal and sinus hygiene with saline rinse/lavage.
- Gently humidify indoor air.
- Use effective nasal steroid sprays.

What to Know About Exercise-Induced Bronchospasm (EIB)

Exercise can be a trigger for many patients with asthma. (If you have respiratory symptoms during or after exercise, see your doctor to make the diagnosis, receive advice and proper treatment, as well as to exclude other medical conditions.) There's a second group that is not asthmatic but suffers asthma symptoms only when exercising. As much as 10 to 15 percent of Americans may suffer from this narrowing of the air passage, a condition called exercise-induced bronchospasm (EIB).

A major factor in EIB may be the tendency for athletes to breathe through the mouth, not nose, during strenuous activity. This is physiologically less desirable: You prevent the nasal passages from filtering, warming, and humidifying air before it's sent down to the lungs. Warmer, moister air is easier on the lungs than cold, dry air, hence the greater chance of triggering asthma symptoms. (This is why exercising in cold, even for non-asthmatics, may lead to chest pain: The outside air is still cold and dry when it hits the airways.) Typical symptoms include cough, chest tightness, wheezing, and reduced fitness capacity. Activities more likely to trigger, or worsen, asthma are marked by constant strenuousness, such as basketball, long-distance running, skating, hockey, and cross-country skiing. Activities less likely to trigger EIB include walking, noncompetitive cycling, swimming, baseball, downhill skiing, football, short-distance track and field, and golf.

EIB typically kicks in around three minutes after exercise begins and peaks at about fifteen minutes. It generally resolves within an hour. To prevent or modify symptoms of EIB:

1. Warm up with low-level exercise, stretching for five to fifteen minutes before the start of the activity.
2. During winter, use a face mask or cotton scarf to help warm and humidify outdoor, cold, and/or dry air before it enters the lungs.
3. Drink water before, during, and after the workout.
4. Complete the workout with a low-key cooldown.
5. Take prescription asthma medicine—often a short-acting, bronchodilator inhaler—fifteen to thirty minutes before the physical activity.

Allergic-Type Asthma

If you're allergic, exposure to substances such as pollen, mold, house dust mite, pet dander, and other allergens will trigger symptoms. If you're asthmatic on top of that, then exposure to these allergens may compromise the airways of the lungs. In allergic asthma, when your immune system responds to various allergens, a host of symptoms, such as swelling and inflammation around the airways, a flooding of mucus, and a triggering of classic asthma symptoms like coughing, wheezing, or shortness of breath, may ensue. (For some people, food and drug allergies can also cause asthma symptoms.)

This is known as allergic asthma (or allergy-induced asthma). By definition, to have allergic asthma is to have both asthma and allergy. It means that your asthma is at least some of the time triggered or worsened by allergens. Allergic asthma is the most common form of asthma: Roughly half of all adults with asthma, as well as 80 to 90 percent of asthmatic kids, have the allergic kind. Symptoms of allergic asthma are similar to those of non-allergic asthma. Less common triggers for allergic asthma include tobacco smoke, smoke from burning wood or grass, air pollution, perfume or other scented products, other strong odors or fumes, air that's cold and dry, changes in the weather, occupational exposures, viral and bacterial infections (e.g., the common cold, sinusitis), acid reflux, some medications (e.g., aspirin or other NSAIDs such as ibuprofen and beta-blockers), exercise, intense emotion (that makes you cry or laugh), and stress. Asthma attacks can be unpredictable and range from mild to moderate to serious to life-threatening.

Asthma's Gender Bias

Although asthma affects boys more than girls, by adulthood the balance has shifted. In the United States, roughly 9 percent of females have asthma versus just under 6.5 percent of males; by age forty, asthma risk for women is double that of men. More women die from it. My colleagues and I have seen an increase among women in asthmatic severity, ER visits, hospitalizations, and mortality; we don't yet know why. Some researchers suspect that hormones associated with the reproductive cycle and/or hormone replacement therapy may increase the risk of severe asthma.

WHO'S AT RISK?

How do you know if your condition is allergic asthma rather than something else? After all, respiratory conditions may appear to be allergic asthma but aren't—for example, it may be occupational asthma, which is triggered by workplace irritants in high concentration, or respiratory hypersensitivity, where dust, mold, chemicals, and other substances trigger a response in the respiratory tract.

If you have hay fever or other allergies, your risk for asthma is heightened. If you have a family history of allergy, your risk for allergic asthma is heightened. Your doctor will want a rundown of other pertinent clues: Breathing issues, other lung conditions in the family, and the prevalence of eczema are also red flags.

An in-office skin prick test—or, if that's not possible, then a blood test—can help to determine the likelihood that you may have an allergy.

For those age twelve and older, there's a simple way to assess your current asthma situation. Ask your asthma specialist or health care provider for an Asthma Control Test (ACT), which generates a better understanding of your condition. The ACT evaluates your symptoms, using a scale from 0 (totally controlled) to 6 (severely uncontrolled) on seven questions, concerning symptoms during the day; symptoms at night; possible limitations of activity; airway caliber; and rescue bronchodilator use. The test is designed to spur discussion with your provider, and help determine the best steps to rein in symptoms. A total score of 19 or lower indicates that your asthma is not properly controlled.

Children often outgrow their wheezing and asthma. However, if your child has eczema or allergies, a pronounced family history of asthma or allergy, and/or there's smoking in the home, the risk is increased that her asthma will continue into adulthood.

As much as it's up to you to determine your environment and behaviors, I can't emphasize this enough: *Do not allow anyone to smoke in your home.*[1]

---

1. Smoking for recreational use—i.e., marijuana—is discouraged, even more so for those with asthma and respiratory disease.

TREATMENT

Because it is a chronic disease, asthma necessitates continual vigilance. By managing allergy, bouts of allergic asthma can be diminished in both frequency and severity. We tailor the approach, which potentially includes a mix of multiple drugs, pharmaceutical *and* biological compounds, and environmental modifications.

Knowing if your asthma is the allergic type is hugely helpful, because daily medications can address allergy symptoms *and* asthma symptoms. Some medicines are inhaled, some taken in pill form. Some are for daily use, some less frequently, some to be taken over a period of years. Medications we may use:

- *Quick-relief medicine,* or a bronchodilator, is known as "rescue medication": It provides temporary symptom relief and is vital during an asthma attack. This medicine is not designed for daily intake except possibly as pretreatment before exercise. It may be given through an inhaler or nebulizer machine. Its purpose is to relax the muscles around the lung's airways, enabling less labored breathing. If you're taking rescue medication more than twice weekly, speak with your doctor.

- *Long-term controller medication* is designed to handle frequent symptoms; it is taken daily. It controls airway inflammation associated with asthma and curtails symptoms. Inhaled corticosteroids are an example of this medicine; they are the most effective anti-inflammatory controller medication available. Leukotriene modifiers are used as an oral tablet to treat and/or prevent asthma. Long-acting bronchodilators may be combined with inhaled corticosteroids to prevent symptoms, and for long-term control of moderate or severe persistent asthma. Like other medicines, asthma drugs have side effects. Discuss with your doctor the intended benefits of all asthma medicines, as well as the risks and possible side effects.

- *Anti-immunoglobulin E (IgE) medication* (*biologics*) reduces the

IgE antibody produced by the immune system. There's clear evidence that anti-IgE therapy can be effective, as an addition to other asthma drugs, in reducing the rate of asthma complications, inhaled corticosteroid dose, and the need for rescue medication in patients with allergic asthma. This medicine is given by injection, usually once or twice monthly, and helps manage symptoms of those whose allergic asthma is moderate to severe.

- *Anti IL agents* for severe asthma. Some are now approved and available in the United States; more are on the way. They appear to be effective, in selected patients, in reducing symptoms and exacerbations of asthma.

- *Allergy shots (immunotherapy)* have shown benefit in some individuals with allergic asthma. The aim is to gradually lower the immune system's reaction to known allergy triggers; this has been shown to reduce asthma symptoms, decrease medication use, and have a favorable effect on bronchial hyper-responsiveness. Immunotherapy may also be referred to as "desensitization." With injection therapy or SCIT (subcutaneous immunotherapy), short-lived localized skin reactions are common; generalized reactions, including anaphylaxis, can occur.

As mentioned earlier, allergy management is guided by four principles, and the first two, avoidance and environmental/behavior modification, are key to asthma management as well. It's critical to feel comfortable in your environment—but how? By avoiding triggers; by remediating the environment at home (see chapter 6 for much more on that); at work (though it's challenging to remove triggers from a space that's not entirely yours to modify); for kids with asthma, at school (the American Lung Association's Open Airways for Schools program educates kids on asthma self-management) and camp (the Consortium for Children's Asthma Camps shares information on controlling triggers, as well as creating a comfortable environment away from home).

When I work with asthmatic patients, we devise an "asthma action plan," with four goals: understand the condition, know what to do if asthma flares, prevent an attack (as much as possible), and improve communication with those around you.

Joey, a ten-year-old boy from Washington Heights in Manhattan, has a history of pet allergies and moderate asthma, and lives in an apartment building loaded with cats and dogs. What's the asthma action plan for him and his family?

- Make a list of the symptoms to watch for: coughing, wheezing, trouble breathing, and chest tightness resulting from exposure to pets and exercise.
- Write up instructions on the type of asthma medication he requires, and usage and dosage for each. On Tuesdays and Thursdays, when he has gym, remind him to take premedication to curb respiratory symptoms.
- Have a written plan ready, right on the refrigerator door, for how to treat Joey's asthma flare-ups.
- Make sure Joey himself knows the steps to take, and when to seek urgent- and emergency-level care.

This action plan enables optimal communication about Joey's asthma management between him and his loved ones. Incredibly, reports indicate that slightly less than half of asthmatic adults have an asthma action plan spelled out; worse, less than one-third of asthmatic children do!

Allergy symptoms change, as do asthma symptoms; ergo, so do allergic asthma symptoms. Adjust treatment to accommodate variations. If symptoms become more severe, other meds may be needed. The number one best thing you can do: *Avoid known allergic triggers*. After you and your doctor consult on an asthma action plan, write down/record the details, as above: This plan—especially the emergency information—should be shared with loved ones and colleagues, just in case.

Anaphylaxis

I see patients almost every day who have experienced a frightening episode of anaphylaxis. In fact, one reason I became an allergist, and view my job as part-sleuth, is to figure out the likely triggers behind this severe, rapid-onset, potentially life-threatening condition and to help devise a way to prevent it from affecting the patient in the future. Here is the simplest way to think about anaphylaxis. Good management of this potential condition means being:

- educated about ways to reduce exposure
- aware of the warning signs and symptoms—i.e., writing up an "action plan"
- prepared to react promptly and correctly, in the unlikely event that it happens

Anaphylaxis (or anaphylactic reaction or anaphylactic shock) is thought to occur in 2 percent of the population, though a recent nationwide survey, "Anaphylaxis in America," identified up to 8 percent of respondents who reported a personal history of anaphylaxis. It is an allergic response—an *over*-over-response, really, compared to most allergic responses—to insect sting, food, medication or latex. Though these are rare, anaphylaxis may occur in response to exercise, or during/after exercise that follows the eating of an allergenic food; or with no identifiable trigger (idiopathic anaphylaxis).

While a "normal" allergic reaction usually locates in one part of the body—e.g., nasal allergies—anaphylaxis may attack one or more areas, including the skin, respiratory, gastrointestinal, and cardiovascular systems. A mixture of symptoms—swelling of lips, throat, eyelids; breathing difficulty, dizziness, fainting, confusion; drop in blood pressure; hives, itching, rash; cramps, nausea, vomiting—is the norm. Anxiety and headache may also be symptoms.

Those with allergies or asthma, or with a family history of anaphylaxis, are at heightened risk for this extreme reaction. Anaphylaxis, which is highly unpredictable, should be treated immediately and properly; it can result in death. (There are no accurate data in the United States for annual fatalities due to anaphylaxis.)

In the event of anaphylaxis, a companion should:

- Call 911 or the local emergency number.
- Use the patient's epinephrine auto-injector; instructions are noted on the device. Epinephrine should be given immediately, within minutes.
- The patient should be sitting or lying down, except if there is trouble with breathing or vomiting.
- Loosen tight-fitting clothing.
- If there are people nearby, ask for assistance.
- If patient has asthma, consider a prescription rescue inhaler (if needed).
- Consider oral antihistamines following epinephrine.
- Remain calm while awaiting medical assistance.
- Transport to ER as soon as possible.
- Always be prepared to give a second dose of epinephrine, if needed.

The person should be taken to a hospital emergency room (by EMS), even if the worst of the episode has passed, for evaluation and further possible treatment. It's important to manage postrecovery, particularly consulting with a doctor to help understand what might have caused the reaction and to protect against future episodes.

If you are highly allergic, have in place an emergency action plan that includes an epinephrine auto-injector and a detailed understanding by your close circle of the potential situation *before* anything happens.

Eyes

The eyes may be the window to the soul; they are also, unfortunately, one of the most visible sites for inflammation due to allergy. The mast cell—the main cell that produces the body's allergic response—is in abundance in the conjunctiva, the mucous membrane covering the white part of the eye and lining the inner eyelid; 50 million mast cells reside there. When the conjunctiva get inflamed, we call it ocular allergy or allergic conjunctivitis. Eyes become itchy, painful, red, and watery.

In summer, eyes-only symptoms are more common than nose-only. Five of every six people who suffer from allergy report some eye-related symptom. A significant number of Americans suffer at some point from watery or itchy eyes, with half of those calling the disturbance moderate to severe. As much as 20 percent or more of the US population is affected by symptoms of eye allergy, a rate that is rising. In one study, half of all women said that eye-impacted allergies negatively affected their appearance. In the midst of allergy season, an estimated 20 percent of contact lens wearers discontinue their use.

That's a lot of disrupted daily routine. In my practice, I see lots more combination sinus-eye ailments. I see more cases with inflammation of the eye, and more persistent and chronic cases. I often see cases where tearing is severe.

A FEW BASICS

Allergy that primarily or secondarily affects the eyes may be year-round or seasonal. Triggers include outdoor allergens like pollen and (less commonly) outdoor mold, and indoor allergens (e.g., house dust mites, pet dander). Symptoms usually set in quickly after exposure. Or the culprit may not be an allergen and only seem that way.

Symptoms for eye allergy are not contagious—unlike pinkeye, which is highly contagious. In most cases, allergy affects both eyes.

The most common medications for treating eye allergy are antihistamines, both topical (drops) and oral. Dual-action antihistamine–mast cell stabilizing agents (drops) such as olopatadine (Patanol, Pazeo), alcaftadine (Lastacaft), bepotastine (Bepreve), and azelastine HCi (Optivar) often provide first-line relief faster than oral antihistamines. More recently, we recommend topical antihistamine *with* mast-cell stabilizers.

If symptoms persist, especially during a period of high pollen, you may benefit from using these medications for days or weeks, following an examination to determine the best treatment option.

Allergic Conjunctivitis

When aeroallergens (dust, pet dander, pollen) contact the eye surface, IgE antibodies are triggered, leading to inflammation. Eyes turn red and itchy, sometimes burning, with tearing or watery discharge, and swelling of the lid. The most telltale symptom of allergic conjunctivitis is itching of and around the eye.

Seasonal allergic conjunctivitis (SAC) may occur immediately or up to days or weeks following exposure. Acute allergic conjunctivitis comes on suddenly, sometimes within minutes. Perennial allergic conjunctivitis (PAC) also may vary in onset, depending on the volume and duration of allergic exposure. Read more about avoidance and treatment techniques for seasonal/outdoor allergy in chapter 5, and for perennial/indoor allergy in chapter 6. My top two pieces of advice:

- Avoid the offending allergen, where possible.
- Modify your environment (e.g., keep home and car windows closed during peak pollen; use an air-conditioner; limit your outdoor exposure).

When the conjunctiva become red and inflamed, you likely have pinkeye. It is not an allergy but an infection, caused in most cases by a virus; less likely, it's bacterial. Discharge from the eyes is frequently present; the eyelids can be extremely swollen. Pinkeye is frequently associated with a cold or respiratory infection, so you may also notice a swollen lymph node, often in front of the ear.

Pinkeye is highly contagious. Meticulous hand-washing and refraining from sharing towels are important steps to keeping pinkeye from spreading. Since it's usually a virus, there is generally no medication for treating it; bacterial pinkeye may be resolved with antibiotics. An eye infection (acute conjunctivitis) caused by pinkeye virus tends to last for five to seven days but can last for weeks, and even become chronic. Both viral and bacterial infections are contagious but don't present exactly the same: The bacterial kind often features a yellow-green discharge in the corner of the eye, sticky enough to keep the eyelids clamped shut upon waking.

As with other conditions, we diagnose allergic conjunctivitis based on the patient's individual and family health history, as well as signs and symptoms. Itchy eyes are almost always a hallmark; if not, then it's likely not allergic conjunctivitis but another condition.

When allergic conjunctivitis meets rhinitis, it is *allergic rhinoconjunctivitis*—the single most prevalent allergic disease. The menu of symptoms is broader, as one would guess—both ocular (conjunctivitis) and nasal (rhinitis).

Other Types of Conjunctivitis

Many contact lens wearers suffer from allergic conjunctivitis. It's commonly triggered by lens irritation or an allergy (perhaps a bacteria-killing preservative like BAK, for benzalkonium chloride, found in contact lens solution and eye drops, or thimerosal, also an ophthalmic preservative). Ophthalmologists often suggest switching to one-day disposable lenses and preservative-free solution, or perhaps taking a break from wearing lenses.

Eye care practitioners and allergists see cases of giant papillary conjunctivitis (GPC), which also affects those who wear contact lenses (more for soft lenses than hard) and use lens solution. Debris on the lens, or continuous eye rubbing, can lead to irritation. GPC is a more extreme form of allergic conjunctivitis, and may occur even in the absence of allergy. Along with the usual symptoms—itchiness, tearing, mucus discharge—GPC is characterized by sacs of fluid (papules) developing in the inner eyelid's upper lining. The answer, as above, is to switch to disposable daily lenses and do away with your current lens solution.

Atopic Keratoconjunctivitis

This condition tends to affect those with a history of eczema or asthma. Atopy means a genetic, greater-than-normal immune response; "atopic" is sometimes referred to as "hyperallergic." The condition tends to worsen in winter. Symptoms include itching, burning, tearing, photo-phobia (sensitivity to light), and red, hardened eyelids; it tends to affect lower lids more than upper. Peak range of incidence is thirty to fifty years old, and it impacts men more than women.

Vernal Keratoconjunctivitis

This allergy is generally more severe than SAC or PAC; three-quarters of those who have it also have eczema or asthma. Generally seasonal, its peak happens between April and August, tending to affect those more in warm, dry climates. Among the usual ocular symptoms, there is thickening/swelling of the conjunctiva, as well as hard, raised bumps on the upper eyelid.

Dry Eye (Tear Film Insufficiency)

It's possible to mistake an allergic reaction for dry eye, a very common condition. While itching tends to accompany allergic conjunctivitis or other eye allergy, it's also a symptom when debris or some other irritant gets in the eye, producing a gritty, dry feeling. Eyes can also feel dry because of fatigue, sun, or wind.

Other symptoms: stinging or burning, eye discharge, redness, and heavy-feeling eyelids. While blurring is common in moderate to severe dry eye, significant vision impairment is rare.

Dry eye may be triggered by menopause or diseases linked with tear production, like rheumatoid arthritis and lupus. Dry eye may also result

---

Wait, Dry Eye Can Cause . . . Watery Eyes?

◾

With dry eye, you produce tears that are lower in water content. Your (infrequent) tears are blinked away quickly, depriving the eyes of being moistened and feeling normal. The inadequate lubrication of the eye surface leads to more blinking, which signals/warns your system that more lubrication is needed. With your tear-making functioning improperly, a rush of tears—"reflex tearing"—is produced by the lacrimal glands.

---

from medication that decreases the secretion of tears—not just antihistamines and decongestants but also sleeping pills, anti-anxiety medicines, pain relievers, and high-blood-pressure medicines. A dry, windy climate tends to worsen dry eye, as do smoke and air conditioning, which speed up tear evaporation.

Saline lubricant/drops help to maintain moisture balance while reducing tearing. Topical cyclosporine may reduce inflammation, and help a return to equilibrium in tear production. The currently popular medication Restasis is designed to increase tear production.

Some other options include artificial tears solution (usually in drop form, but may also be ointment or gel); artificial tears (such as hydromethylcellulose), an insert to keep the eye moist (a lubricant is placed daily under the lower eye, and release is sustained over the course of the day); and punctal plugs, which stop up the tear ducts, closing off the tiny opening in the inner corner of the lower and upper eyelid and helping to conserve the limited supply of tears you're producing, plus any artificial tears you are adding.

Blepharitis

This common condition results from residual eye drops that spill out of the eye onto the eyelashes, hardening and leaving crust and flakes on the lashes. Symptoms also include itchiness, redness, swelling of the eyelids; dry eyes; and even sensitivity to light and blurred vision. We often see blepharitis in those with rosacea—reddened skin and irritation on the face and eyelids.

Eyelid inflammation and swelling happen for a variety of reasons: infection; insufficient hygiene; blockage of the eyelid's oil glands. My patients who suffer from blepharitis (more women than men) may contract it through their use of eye care and skin cosmetics. Allergies may contribute to blepharitis, too, though the root of the vulnerability may be hormone imbalance.

Care must be taken to clean eyes and lids (loosening clogged oils from the glands behind the lashes) to avoid damage and scarring to eye tissue. You may treat blepharitis with a warm, wet, clean washcloth or a warm compress, as directed by your eye care professional. To help reduce recurrence, remove eye makeup before bed and refrain from applying eyeliner on the eyelid's back edge, behind the eyelashes.

Eyelid Dermatitis

This is often caused by contact with allergens, particularly preservatives and fragrances, found in cosmetics, hair care and nail products, ointments, eye drops, and contact lens solution. Patch testing may identify the culprit.

Before Eye Go

■

If you wear contact lenses, do not apply eye drops. I often recommend that my patient, after having removed her lenses, use a once-daily ocular antihistamine, in eye drop form. It can relieve itchy, watery, and red eyes for up to twenty-four hours. In some cases, dryness may accompany its usage.

Taking the Red Eye

■

Terry, a thirty-one-year-old contact lens wearer, visited our office at the recommendation of her ophthalmologist. Her eyelids were red and puffy, possibly a reaction to one of her eye cosmetics or contact lens solution. She wisely brought in all her eye care products, facial cosmetics, and solutions for evaluation. Testing uncovered two issues: Her skin was highly sensitive to pet dander (her dog and cat both slept on her bed), and she had an allergy to a preservative commonly used in cleaning and refreshing lens solutions. We found her a preservative-free lens cleaning solution, plus other face products free of that preservative, and within days of using those she was looking much better—though not completely resolved. She agreed to consider—*consider*—having the pets sleep somewhere but the bed, though she insisted they would stay in her room.

The Eyes Have It—Up to a Point

■

Over-the-counter decongestant eye drops can reduce redness, but just as I cautioned against using nasal decongestant spray for more than three days because of the risk of rebound nasal congestion, so, too, pharmaceutical manufacturers generally suggest refraining from prolonged use (three or more consecutive days) of this medication. Overuse can lead to eye irritation and reduction in the medication's effectiveness. For dry eyes, moisturizing eye drops can make you feel a little better but will not diminish allergy symptoms.

Chapter 5

Outdoor and Seasonal Allergies

We want to be out in the world, in nature, in the park, in our garden, breathing the air in the beautiful outdoors.

Isn't it pretty to think so?

Roughly 20 percent of allergy sufferers have seasonal, or outdoor, allergies, while another 40 percent suffer from both seasonal and year-round (non-outdoor-specific) allergies. When your immune system overreacts to airborne allergens, you need to regularly excuse yourself from all that inviting greenery. If you could choose between the two kinds of allergy, the preference would seem to be the one "designed" to last only part of the year, often for just a couple of months. To anyone who has it, though, seasonal allergy, particularly seasonal allergic rhinitis, better known as hay fever (aka pollinosis), is no picnic: symptoms include nasal itching/repeated nose rubbing, mouth breathing, itchy eyes, and allergic shiners. That's just the start, though. When it persists, hay fever and other seasonal allergy are often debilitating, restricting your capacity to function well outdoors and partake in many of the vigorous activities that make life joyful.

The presentation of outdoor and indoor allergy are the same; it doesn't matter whether your triggers are pollen, dust mite, or pet dander. The immune mechanism is the same. Researchers explain the nature of the problem (part of it anyway) with a concept called "nasal priming": More pollen (to take the seasonal example) enters the nasal mucosa (membrane) over sequential days, likely triggering a response that builds, so that a flood of inflammatory cells release mediators such as histamine, meaning more severe symptoms. "Priming" basically means enhanced sensitivity/response to the allergen with each exposure: Over time there are more bothersome days. This may explain the perception that your medication is not working as expected. One study showed that nasal symptoms at the end of pollen season were worse than at the start, though the level of ragweed pollen in the air is roughly equal. (Better news: A study from the University of Chicago showed that use of nasal steroid spray can help prevent nasal priming, thus allowing for symptom improvement overall.)

During allergy seasons, symptoms worsen when you're outdoors, and near fresh-cut grass; they tend to improve when you retreat to air-conditioned spaces. It's more a young person's challenge: Many of my patients are under age twenty, though the condition tends not to first appear until after the child is four or five years old because (it's believed) it can take approximately three seasons of pollen exposure before the antibody buildup and subsequent reaction kick in.

Who gets seasonal allergies? Again, family history is a strong determinant, but there are environmental factors, too. Weather changes determine everything from when allergy starts to when it ends to how bad it is to how far-reaching. If you think your hay fever or allergic asthma is worsening over time, you may be right—and it may have little to do with your own physiology. As I noted at the beginning of the book, climate change may increase the length and severity of pollen seasons, leading to increased exposure to allergenic pollens. Shifting weather patterns often mean longer allergic impact, and what once was reasonably called "seasonal" now feels closer to year-round. Due to climate change, our allergenic seasons are now both longer *and* perhaps more potent.

The change is troubling not just for those with hay fever, who may suffer worse symptoms over a more extended period. Longer springs mean more pollen exposure for *everyone*, meaning that those not (yet) allergic may be at greater risk for developing sensitivity and eventually allergy than if they were exposed less to these allergens. Changing weather patterns may be particularly bad for asthmatics: More allergens, and increased ozone pollution, can trigger flare-ups.

How can you best fight seasonal allergy? What are the steps to keep triggers from setting off symptoms? It takes not one life change but rather a seasonal action plan, which includes preventions of the primary, secondary, and tertiary kind. It includes trigger avoidance (espe-

Should I Stay or Should I Go?

Allergy can be so debilitating that patients often wonder if moving to an allergy-friendlier location will solve their problem. Could relocating to a different part of the country help to reduce the frequency, severity and duration of symptoms? Perhaps—but maybe not. Numerous types of pollen, particularly grasses, and molds are found in most "plant zones" (regions defined by their annual minimum winter temperature, on average). So regional upheaval may not yield the desired result, especially since warming climate has affected all parts of the country (if not equally), meaning a longer spring-summer "season" elsewhere, meaning a greater barrage of pollen and mold spores generally.

Suppose a move does bring relief from allergens that were abundant in your previous environment. There's no guarantee that allergens indigenous to your new home won't become triggers. Several patients told me that they moved more than a thousand miles away from their previous home, and it did have a beneficial effect, for about seven or eight years—after which they developed allergy to the culprits in their (relatively) new environment.

And one more thing. Because pollen can travel hundreds of miles via wind, your reaction may be to plants that aren't even in your local environment!

cially during peak pollen), environmental modification, and overall "allergy alertness." While I advocate for less pharmacotherapy where possible, OTC medication plays an important role in short-term relief, while immunotherapy—allergy shots—may provide lasting symptom remission, or an "allergy time-out," and help to prevent the development of new allergies and asthma. You may benefit from a visit to an allergist or ENT doctor.

Let's get to the specifics of seasonal allergy, and what can be done about it.

The Pollen Predicament—or, What Seasons We Mean When We Say "Seasonal Allergy"

Pollen grains are male reproductive cells produced by trees, weeds, plants, and grasses, released to fertilize the female part of the plant, leading to the development of new seed. Pollen is produced only by male flowers, or the male parts of flowers. Some plant species fertilize themselves, while others cross-pollinate: The pollen is transmitted from the flower of one plant to another flower of the same species. To reach its destination, pollen usually travels via insect or wind (birds and water are also conveyors). The warmer the locale, the longer the pollination cycle; in certain warm locations, pollination may be year-round. Each pollen grain may be functionally "viable" for only a few minutes to a few hours (the hotter and sunnier the day, the briefer the time it's viable); unfortunately for us, its capacity to trigger allergic reaction can go on and on.

Not all pollens are created equal. Depending on the plant and region it inhabits, the size, weight, and moisture content of pollen will vary. This, along with the weather, affects how long pollen remain airborne. Pollen are microscopic, often round or oval in shape, often in powdery form; a pollen grain, on average, is 20 microns in diameter. (Imagine those square holes that make up the mesh in a screen on a window or door: About one thousand grains, simultaneously, could slip through one square.) The smaller the pollen, the more easily inhaled. Smaller pollen may trigger a stronger response because the grains can penetrate deeper into the lungs. The reaction, and its severity, may also be influenced by the particular proteins on the pollen's surface.

Heavier pollen often falls to the ground, near its plant of origin. Such plants rarely cause allergy for the simple reason that their pollen isn't airborne, hence not nearly as inhalable, and it doesn't scatter.

When pollen is especially small, light, and dry, it can travel via wind for extraordinary distances: Ragweed pollen has been measured at over 10,000 feet in the air, and 400 miles out to sea.

Typically, the most allergenic pollen comes from plants that do not sport "showy" flowers—trees, grasses and weeds, which produce prodigious amounts of pollen. (A single ragweed plant can produce up to a billion pollen grains in one season.) Their pollen tends to be light and dry, ideal for being carried significant distances by wind. These plants are a big problem for the allergic.

How does pollen then get inside the home? Via windows and heating and cooling vents—or it often walks right in through the door. For example, bottlebrush produces triangular pollen, which does not travel well in the air but sticks easily to a dog's fur; when inhaled, it's one of the most explosively allergenic triggers around—and the family dog may be the source of exposure for everyone in the home.

Don't Suppose It's Roses

If you're seasonally allergic, you may believe you're vulnerable primarily to flowers that are scented or colorful, such as roses—but that's unlikely. The pollen grains for such plants tend to be bigger, heavier and waxy, and get ferried to other plants/flowers by bees, butterflies, and other insects, not wind.

The reaction to such fragrant, beautiful plants is more commonly an irritation to the eyes and nasal passages, not allergy.

Allergy Seasons in Areas of the Country
with Three or Four Seasons

Spring: During the first weeks, trees begin releasing pollen. Some key offenders: alder, ash, birch, box elder, cottonwood, non-American elm, hickory, maple, mountain cedar, juniper, mulberry, oak, and pecan.

Late spring/summer: Grass pollen fills the air in April/early May through mid-July. It's hay fever season. Weeds may begin pollination during spring, perhaps later. There are over one thousand species of North American grasses but certain varieties are notably allergenic: Bermuda, fescue, Johnson, Kentucky bluegrass (June grass), orchard grass, redtop, rye, sweet vernal, and Timothy.

Late summer/fall: Most weeds, including ragweed, produce their pollen, and may continue doing so until first frost. Pollen is also produced by English plantain, lamb's quarters, redroot pigweed, sagebrush, and tumbleweed (Russian thistle). "Southern" grasses such as Bermuda and Johnson are at their peak.

The seasons outlined above are approximations. In certain locales, especially in the South and Southwest, pollination may occur throughout the year, or start at different times, or may produce and release pollen in greater volume than in other regions. In much of Texas, pollination from male mountain cedars (not a true cedar but a species of juniper) begins around Christmas. In the West and South, where winters may be mild, landscape trees and shrubs can bloom year-round. In the Pacific Northwest, hay fever season may feature up to ten times the airborne grass pollen typically released in other regions. In California, the state that produces the most olives, olive tree pollen can be unbearable for those who drive by orchards; olive pollen is a frequent trigger of allergy and asthma. (Some Southwestern cities, such as Tucson, Las Vegas, Albuquerque, and El Paso, have Pollen Control Ordinances forbidding the sale or planting of any more olive trees.) The northern United States has experienced significant weather changes, with pollen now traveling greater distances than it once did. So changes in (short-term) weather and (long-term) climate, along with other variables, profoundly influence the start date, end date, and severity of allergy seasons.

Keep in mind:

- Rainfall tends to suppress airborne pollen (though during thunderstorms and afterward, the opposite may be true—see "Thunderstorm Asthma," page 94). Pollen is washed to the ground, where it's less inhalable.
- Mold count rises, generally, with precipitation.
- When combined with air pollutants, especially ground-level ozone, airborne allergens lead to more, and more severe, allergy symptoms. Certain trees are large net producers of BVOCs— biogenic volatile organic compounds, particularly ground-level ozone. Eucalyptus and oak trees are among the worst offenders. Planting such trees in urban areas does nothing to improve air quality, much less alleviate allergy.
- Pollen dispersed by wind extends the region of exposure.
- Particularly at northern latitudes, snowfall may delay the onset of flowering, meaning a later start to allergy season. In some areas, in certain years, a very late, hard frost kills all the male flowers on male trees such as cottonwood, poplar, willow, etc., before they release any pollen, leading to a much lower pollen level.

The population of hay fever sufferers is not evenly distributed. This map shows variations in types of hay fever around the United States.

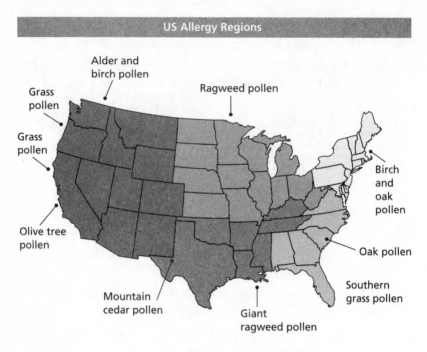

US Allergy Regions

Alder and birch pollen

Grass pollen

Grass pollen

Ragweed pollen

Olive tree pollen

Birch and oak pollen

Oak pollen

Mountain cedar pollen

Giant ragweed pollen

Southern grass pollen

National Allergy Bureau; American Academy of Allergy, Asthma, and Immunology

And the map on the opposite page shows how the concentration of a given allergen source—in this case, Kentucky bluegrass—varies from region to region.

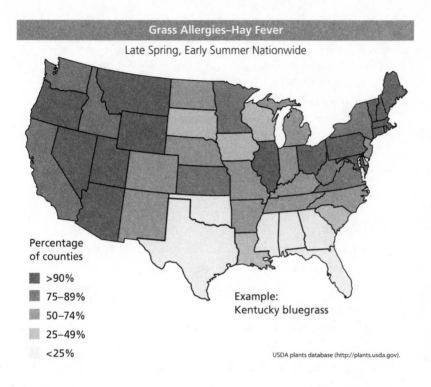

Grass Allergies–Hay Fever

Late Spring, Early Summer Nationwide

Percentage
of counties

■ >90%

■ 75–89%

■ 50–74%

25–49%

<25%

Example:
Kentucky bluegrass

USDA plants database (http://plants.usda.gov).

Pollen Count vs. Pollen Forecast

■

Helpfully, the National Allergy Bureau (NAB), part of the American Academy of Allergy, Asthma, and Immunology's (AAAAI) Aeroallergen Network, measures the air's pollen and mold content in given areas. "Pollen count" is a real-time number for what's out there now: The figure is the measurement of pollen grains per square meter of air, collected over twenty-four hours. "Pollen forecast" (or "mold forecast") is a prediction based on existing data of pollen/mold and weather in the given region/ time frame.

Sign up for a personalized e-mail alert from the NAB (aaaai .org/nab), which reports reliable pollen/mold levels for five regions of the United States and Canada, courtesy of nearly eighty "counting" stations throughout those countries. Or get the AAAAI's pollen app by using your mobile device to go to pollen.aaaai.org.

Smart Steps

- Limit outdoor activities during peak pollen times and/or plan ahead with a proactive approach to managing your allergies—for example, by premedicating before outdoor activities.
- Keep windows closed, when possible.
- Air-conditioning cleans and dries air. Wash or change the AC filter regularly.
- Eliminate the most allergenic trees and shrubs from your yard; replace them with allergy-friendly substitutes. (Read about the Ogren Pollen Allergy Scale [OPALS] on page 99.)
- When outdoors, wear sunglasses (bigger means better coverage) and a hat. If you must be outdoors doing things like mowing and weeding for an extended period, wear a pollen mask. (Also known as a dust mask or respirator, the mask comes in three classes: FFP1, FFP2, and FFP3, with increasingly impenetrable filters. An FFP2 dust mask, for instance, filters out a minimum of 94 percent of airborne particles, and lets in less than 8 percent. Get a mask with an exhalation valve to make breathing out potentially less laborious.)
- When you return home, shower. Use a facecloth to clean eyelid margins safely and properly. Shampoo nightly.
- Change clothes, particularly before entering your bedroom.
- Try to avoid line-drying sheets or clothes outdoors.
- When in cars, keep windows closed (at least during pollen season). Use the air conditioner.
- Follow instructions for prescribed/recommended medications.

Tree Sexism—and Why We Need a More Female Arboreal Presence

Trees that produce few or no fruits or nuts are easier to clean up. City governments and store owners like that. Nurseries often like that. The problem? While such trees shed few leaves or flowers, they most certainly produce pollen, and tend to be highly allergenic. And many of these "litter-free" trees tend to be male.

Roughly half a century ago, the tree population in US cities mostly mirrored the natural tree-gender balance in the countryside. Then, partly because of this desire to make cleanup easier, the era of "botanical sexism" was born—and we're still in it. Many female seedlings were removed. Male seedlings remained, and male "clones" of separate-sexed trees (which produce no seeds but lots more pollen than dual-sexed trees) abounded—ash, box elder, cypress, juniper, maple, mulberry, olive, podocarpus, yew. (Most olive varieties produce both male and female flower parts.) The far less messy, far more allergenic male trees proliferated. With the scourge of Dutch elm disease, this trend increased: Wherever dying trees were replaced with more allergenic male clones, pollen allergy increased—first along the East Coast; then, by a decade and a half later, along the West Coast.

The dearth of female trees hurts the allergy sufferer a second way: Female flowers generate a slightly negative charge; pollen, as it floats through air, develops a charge that's slightly positive. The female flower would attract the pollen, in effect cleaning the air of it . . . rather than letting the noses of allergy sufferers do the job.

"THUNDERSTORM ASTHMA"—THE STORM
BEFORE THE (NOT) CALM

The baseball game was delayed to let a thunderstorm pass. A violent storm, tons of rain—then blue skies. The game started. A boy with asthma and allergy, who I've seen at my practice, hit a ball between the outfielders but had trouble running the bases. Soon, he was wheezing, appeared short of breath, and needed his rescue bronchodilator inhaler before recovering. Was it just his usual asthma, if a bad bout of it? Or something else? Why are there reports of a spike in emergency room visits for worsening asthma during or after a thunderstorm, particularly during pollen season?

When it rains or turns humid, pollen grains can absorb moisture until finally they burst ("pollen rupture"), releasing hundreds of small, potentially allergenic particles that can penetrate deep into the small airways of the lungs, prompting allergy symptoms; for asthmatics, the air during or after a thunderstorm or rain shower can trigger severe symptoms. Mold spores can also burst, unleashing a greater concentration of allergens.

Interestingly, it's not the rain torrent that's behind this phenomenon but really the airflow. The downdraft of cold air concentrates pollen and mold spores; the draft pushes that concentrated air up to heavily humid clouds, where pollen and spores fracture; the allergen shower, in microscopic form, is dispersed by the rain. July may be a particularly bad month, as thunderstorm season couples with a rise in concentration of fungal mold spores, plus a still-ample supply of grass pollen. Research shows that the air in a thunderstorm carries a concentration of grass pollen four to twelve times normal counts.

Your Garden, Your Nose

If you love gardening, your seasonal allergy needn't keep you from it. Immersion in greenery, along with getting hands dirty, are essential, sensory, even joyful aspects to gardening, but they can also mean sneezing, itchy eyes, congestion, and other unpleasant or prohibitive symptoms. To reduce or eliminate the distress:

- Garden when pollen levels are lower. Avoid early mornings, when pollen counts tend to be higher; embrace, especially, days that are rainy, cloudy and/or windless.
- Control weeds; ask someone not allergic to do the job. Have them mow the lawn and rake leaves, activities that whip up pollen and mold.
- Mulch from wood chips retains moisture, which can lead to mold growth. Alternative mulch options: oyster shell, gravel, special plant ground covers like pachysandra or vinca.
- Hedges mean tangled branches that more easily collect pollen, dust, and mold. Prune and thin hedges.
- Cut grass low (around two inches), which limits stems from spreading pollen.
- When doing yard work, try not to touch your eyes or face.
- Wear allergy-protective gear—gloves, goggles, a NIOSH-approved face mask to reduce breathing in pollen spores.[1]
- Keep your home's windows closed during mowing and for some hours afterward.
- Gardening tools and clothing, particularly gloves and shoes, should be left outdoors.
- Shower immediately after gardening.
- Don't wait until symptoms start: If you're on allergy medication, take it preemptively.

A NEW GARDEN MIX

For better breathing and enjoyment of your passion, do more than just follow allergy-smart gardening tactics: The composition of your garden

---

1. The National Institute for Occupational Safety and Health.

matters, too. Cultivate at least some allergy-friendly, or -friendlier, plants, flowers, and trees. Female-only plants produce no pollen. Some plants are more than just less or non-allergenic: When cultivated indoors (especially), they actually "scrub" the air to a possibly beneficial extent. (See chapter 6 for a list of these plants, as identified by NASA.)

Color, fragrance, size, and shape may help to determine how allergenic a plant is. As a rule, small plant flowers with less bright, nondescript colors are likelier to be wind-pollinated, hence likelier to be allergenic. Plants that produce big and/or colorful, fragrant flowers are less likely to have a high allergenic component. Why? As I mentioned earlier, plants with heavier pollen (meaning the pollen is less likely to be airborne, and therefore less likely to be inhaled) rely largely on insects to transport pollen; the more fragrant and floral, the likelier they draw attention as food/nectar sources.

Also, it's wise to keep fragrant night-blooming plants and flowers—for example, moonflower, evening stock, night-blooming jasmine, eucalyptus, primrose, and night-flowering wild petunia—away from open windows; their proximity may worsen symptoms while you're sleeping.

ALLERGIC-FRIENDLY GARDENING CHOICES

- Apple tree
- Asiatic lily
- Azalea
- Begonia
- Bird of Paradise
- Bougainvillea
- Boxwood (if clipped often)
- Bradford pear tree
- Buffalo grass (female clone)
- Cactus
- Camellia
- Clematis
- Columbine
- Crepe myrtle tree

- Crocus
- Cyclamen
- Dahlia (fully double)
- Dianthus
- Dogwood tree
- Dusty Miller
- English holly tree (the females—with berries—are pollen-free)
- Fern pine tree (female)
- Geranium
- Hardy rubber tree
- Heuchera (coralbells)
- Hibiscus
- Hosta
- Hyacinth
- Hydrangea
- Impatiens
- Iris
- Lupine
- Magnolia tree
- Orchid
- Pansy
- Pear tree
- Penstemon
- Periwinkle
- Petunia
- Phlox
- Plum tree
- Podocarpus, fern pine, yew pine (fruiting females are pollen-free)
- Red maple tree (female selections are pollen-free)
- Rose (florist type: hybrid tea, unscented)
- Saint Augustine grass
- Salvia
- Sedum
- Snapdragon

- Thrift
- Tulip (wear gloves when handling bulbs)
- Verbena
- Viburnum
- Viola
- Zinnia (not recommended as a cut flower indoors)

. . . AND NOT-SO-ALLERGIC-FRIENDLY GARDENING CHOICES

- Artemisia
- Ash (male)
- Aster (double ones are much less allergenic)
- Baby's breath (single flower may be a problem, double-flowered variety's a better choice)
- Bluegrass
- Chamomile
- Chrysanthemum (double forms are much less allergenic)
- Dahlia (single flower)
- Fescue
- Gardenia (fragrant)
- Gerber daisy (fine in the garden, allergenic as a cut flower)
- Jasmine (fragrant)
- Johnson grass
- Juniper (male)
- Lavender (fragrant)
- Lilac (fragrant)
- Lily (fragrant, pollen stains, and sap—Peruvian variety—may cause rash)
- Maple
- Narcissus (small form of daffodil; the small white-and-yellow ones are extremely fragrant)
- Oak
- Rye grass
- Sunflower (though newer ones, such as "Teddy Bear," are pollen-free)

- Timothy grass
- Utica or nettle (male)

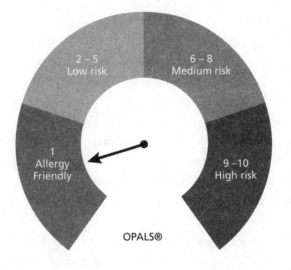

OPALS®

For a more extensive list, horticulturist Tom Ogren has created a standard, the Ogren Plant Allergy Scale (OPALS), which considers the likelihood that a plant—flowers, grasses, shrubs, and trees—will cause pollen allergies, contact allergies, and odor allergies. The OPALS rates the allergy potential of the plant to guide you in reducing your exposure to pollen and irritants that are bothersome, especially if you have allergic sensitivities. His 1–10 scale gives greater consideration to plants that cause pollen allergies due to *inhaling* pollen.

The OPALS ratings can help you or a gardener to create cleaner, less allergenic air and reduce local exposure; those involved with maintenance around elementary and secondary schools to practice allergy-friendly landscaping on school grounds; and housing contractors and landscape designers to create or improve entire neighborhoods with all allergy-friendly plants. Indeed, by using windbreaks of tall trees and tall shrubs, much prevailing wind can be blocked and act as a huge trap for airborne pollen coming from other developments/neighborhoods. The OPALS system has been used by the American Lung Association (which recommends only plants of an OPALS pollen rating of 6 or less) and the USDA Urban Foresters.

Cross-Reaction

Some seasonal allergy may be initiated by a pollen allergy but triggered by food.

Many of my patients refuse to believe their particular problem is caused by a food allergy. Upon further questioning, however, most of them appear to suffer from itchiness of the mouth and throat during and/or after eating many fresh fruits and vegetables such as stone fruit (e.g., plum, cherry, peach), apple, pear, melon, kiwi, carrot, celery, and cucumber, to name some common culprits. Called oral allergy syndrome or pollen-food syndrome, it works like this: You're exposed to pollen protein (likely through inhaling) and develop a sensitization to it, then pollen-specific IgE antibody is manufactured, binding to mast cells and other cells found throughout the body, including the area of the throat behind the mouth.

Then, when you eat certain foods with proteins "related" to the pollen protein due to a structural similarity (homologous), the antibodies "recognize" the food protein (though it's not identical) and trigger a reaction, usually around the mouth and throat area. The mostly localized reaction is not extreme, as the food allergens are soon degraded and rendered harmless once digested. It's estimated that a very, very small percentage of the time, this reaction may morph into a more serious, potentially generalized reaction, not dissimilar to full-blown food allergy. In such a case, an epinephrine auto-injector must be ready to go. My younger sister, Debbie, used to experience mild itchiness in her throat and mouth after eating fresh kiwi. Now? The slightest amount of this fruit is enough to trigger throat irritation and a scary sensation that her throat could "close up."

This phenomenon is called cross-reaction. In springtime, I see quite

It Takes Two (to Cause a Serious Reaction)

Jennifer, a twenty-nine-year-old sales associate, had very bothersome springtime pollen allergy, complete with sneezing attacks, runny nose, and watery, red eyes. She told me that the condition was distracting to her and her customers at the fashion-focused department store where she worked, especially when she was handling pricey apparel and/or jewelry. She noticed that her symptoms gradually worsened, and were complemented by itchiness of the mouth and throat, after her afternoon break, during which she often ate a piece of fruit and had a cup of flavored coffee. In our office, she tested positive for birch pollen allergy, a staple of springtime in New York. But the allergy was made worse by certain foods she consumed—in her case, apple and pears, as well as coffee flavored with real, fresh-ground hazelnut and almond—because they may have cross-reacted with tree pollen. Did she have to give up her favorite fruits? Actually, no: Peeling rendered them harmless to her. And she switched to unflavored coffee. Her seasonal suffering was significantly reduced (though it did not disappear altogether, given her tree pollen allergy). Later, she began a program of allergen immunotherapy and noticed that some of the food-related triggers improved over several months' time.

a few birch tree pollen sufferers whose symptoms worsen upon their eating foods such as apple, pear, or stone fruits that cross-react with the pollen. In summer and fall, I often see cross-reaction in individuals whose ragweed/weed sensitivity is exacerbated by their eating cantaloupe, or other melons, banana, and zucchini (to name a few).

Read more about oral allergy syndrome in chapter 8: Food Allergies.

Poison Ivy

For a detailed discussion of this condition, see chapter 7.

Stinging Insects

If you have insect allergy, you want ways to feel more confident outdoors, and actually be able to enjoy yourself.

If you're *not* allergic to an insect bite or sting, symptoms include redness, itching, and/or swelling at the wound site—not pleasant but not debilitating. Signs of the sting or bite are generally gone in a day or two. If you have developed such an allergy, however, the body's response can be more severe, as the immune system overreacts to the venom. Symptoms include itching, hives, swelling of throat/tongue, breathing difficulty, dizziness, cramps, nausea, vomiting, and unconsciousness.

A reaction beyond the localized area where you were stung or bitten is "insect hypersensitivity." It's not rare that an insect sting results in anaphylaxis. If the reaction is severe, of course, seek emergency care immediately.

What's the best way to deal with venom allergy? First, it helps if you can identify the insects you should be wary of, and the places they call home.

STING OPERATION: KNOW YOUR INSECTS
SO YOU'RE BETTER ABLE TO AVOID THEM[2]

Bumblebees, honeybees: Domesticated honeybees make their homes in human-made hives; the wild variety hole up in honeycombs, found in hollowed trees or spaces in buildings. Provoked, these bees will sting; unbothered, they tend to leave you alone. It's killer bees—actually, Af-

2. Reprinted with permission from the American Academy of Allergy, Asthma, and Immunology, AAAAI.org.

ricanized honeybees, found mostly in the southwest region of the United States—that are more likely to sting, unprovoked, and do so in swarms.

Hornets: Their gray or brown nests are usually set high—in branches, shrubs, tree hollows, gables—shaped like footballs, and built from material like paper.

Yellow jackets: Their papier-mâché-like nests are often found underground but also in woodpiles, masonry cracks, or the walls of buildings. Yellow jackets are smaller than hornets.

Paper wasps: Paperlike material for their nests (note their name) forms a comb of cells in a circle shape that flares toward the ground. Their nests may be found in shrubs, behind shutters, and under leaves.

Fire ants: Typically found in the South/Southeast United States, their dirt nests are built into the ground, frequently at the edge of the road or sidewalk. When their homes are built in sandy, dry soil, they are flat; when built in claylike, moist soil, the mounds reach more than a foot high. The ants do not clear vegetation from their surroundings, making them hard to see.

While it's easy to recommend steering clear of such insects, it's impractical advice for those who like the outdoors and wish to live freely. To reduce risk when outdoors while stinging insects are moving all about:

- Calmly move away.
- Nests around your home should be (sad to say) destroyed—or, if possible, removed.
- Food smells—cooking, sweet drinks (e.g., juice, soda)—may draw insects. Watch for insects lurking inside canned drinks or straws. Until you're hungry, keep food under wraps.
- Wear closed-toe shoes when you're outdoors. And no loose-fitting garments, which may unwittingly ensnare insects.

Wait—What's a Sting and What's a Bite?

■

A sting means that toxic venom has been injected into your system via the insect's, well, stinger. A bite means that anticoagulant saliva has been injected, enabling the insect to consume your blood. Stingers include bees, yellow jackets, wasps, hornets, and fire ants.

Biters include mosquitoes, ticks, fleas, lice, bedbugs, chiggers, and scabies.

TREATING STINGS

Reducing risk is one thing; eliminating it is another. In the presence of stinging insects, remain calm and brush any from your skin. Leave the area quickly. If you've been stung:

- If the stinger remains, remove it from your skin immediately to prevent influx of more venom. You can usually dislodge the stinger and sac with a scrape of your fingernail. Try to not squeeze the sac, which could give you another burst of venom.
- To reduce pain and swelling, raise the stung limb and apply a cold compress.
- Clean the affected area gently with water and soap; this can prevent secondary infection. If there's a blister, do not break it.
- To relieve itchiness, apply topical OTC steroid cream or ointment, or take an oral non-sedating antihistamine (e.g., loratadine, fexofenadine, etc.). For greater potency and effectiveness, your steroid cream may require a prescription.
- If swelling continues or worsens, or if the sting site appears infected, contact your physician.

A small percentage of venom-allergic people can suffer anaphylaxis, and should always carry auto-injectable epinephrine. Epinephrine is a rescue medication only; if stung, you must still take an immediate, accompanied trip to the ER.

Venom immunotherapy is currently the most effective type of immunotherapy. After a successful course of treatment, the risk of a generalized allergic reaction or anaphylaxis is 5 percent or lower.

UBIQUITO: THE EVER-PRESENT MOSQUITO

Is there a scary disease the mosquito does *not* transmit? This small fly is known to carry blood-borne diseases such as malaria, dengue fever, West Nile virus, chikungunya, and now, troublingly, Zika. The vast number of times we notice mosquitoes, though, it's because of their nonserious but extremely nasty bite—or, usually, many bites.

A mosquito bite engenders a range of bodily reactions. For those who have never been bitten, including many young children, there can be no reaction, immediate or delayed, after a mosquito bite. For those who have been bitten before, the reaction is typically a very small, itchy red bump that appears minutes to hours to days after the bite, and which may last a few days. Less commonly, mosquito bite reactions go big. I have dozens of patients with this complaint: They develop red, itchy, painful swelling, which can be mistaken for a bacterial skin infection, cellulitis, and they often get treated at an urgent care facility for this "infection" when it's really a large, protuberant, localized skin reaction. This condition, termed Skeeter syndrome, is an allergic response to the mosquito salivary protein, which progresses over eight or more hours and resolves over days. It may require first aid and medical treatment to hasten its resolution.

When the female mosquito bites (generally, male mosquitoes don't), the tip of her mouth inserts into a tiny blood vessel, saliva gets injected into the bloodstream, and she feeds on the blood. Her saliva contains chemicals that keep human blood from clotting, which in turn causes a response: localized redness, swelling, itching. If contact is under six seconds, a reaction won't occur.

Are mosquitoes ever truly avoidable, given their tiny size and, during parts of the year, ubiquitousness? Not totally. But I have found that my "Stop the Bite" action plan I discuss with my patients helps, enabling them to better enjoy their time outdoors.

1. Take an OTC or prescription oral antihistamine during the "biting" months.
2. Review insect-repellent options; go to cdc.gov or consumerreports .org for up-to-date information.
3. Apply your chosen insect repellent.
4. Use topical OTC cortisone-type cream for mild redness, itchiness, etc.
5. Try ice compresses to reduce inflammation and discomfort.
6. If your reaction is severe or you believe you may have an infection, seek medical attention.

The point is, whether you're non-allergic, mildly allergic, or seriously allergic, you can reduce the chance of a bite. Some other thoughts:

• Dusk to dawn is peak mosquito time. Stay indoors, when possible.
• Avoid shaded, humid, calm areas, as well as pools of standing water—both locales that mosquitoes love.
• How you dress affects how much mosquitoes are drawn to you. The (biting) female is attracted by light, heat, sweat, body odor, lactic acid, and carbon dioxide. It's advisable to wear clothes that cover the majority of your skin (though I realize that it may not be fashionable).
• When outside, wear socks and closed-toe shoes; barefoot is asking for it. While gardening or doing yard work, wear gloves.

Outdoor Mold

The symptoms for allergy to mold or related fungi are similar to those for other seasonal allergy: sneezing; runny nose; nasal congestion; itching of the nose, throat, and oral cavity; and itchy, watery eyes. So how can you know if your allergy is specific to outdoor mold? An allergist can perform a scratch test, in which a small amount of mold allergen is introduced via a very light scratch on your skin; presence of mold sensitivity is confirmed by localized itching, redness, and/or swelling.

What is mold? It is usually a fungus related to yeasts and mushrooms but different from plants in that it lacks stems, roots, flowers, or leaves. Molds can live anywhere that has moisture, and get nourishment from the living and dead materials on plants and animals. As they grow, mold spores react chemically so that they can consume nutrients and multiply; during these chemical reactions, fumes are released (this is the cause of the musty odor associated with mold). The mold spore, its seed, travels through the air no matter the weather: It can disperse when conditions are dry and windy; or, in highly humid conditions, spread in fog or dew.

Molds proliferate with the onset of spring, as temperatures rise, and peak in late summer and into fall, when trees shed their leaves in bulk and plants start to die off. Mold allergy season runs approximately from mid-summer through early autumn. (Indoor mold is a year-round story; see chapter 6.) Throughout the warmer United States (South, West Coast), mold spores peak around July, but may be found year-round; in colder regions, molds peak around October. However, molds, unlike pollen, do not die with the first winter frost (and their allergic potential may remain for a while): For the most part, they simply become inactive. Molds are everywhere, flourishing in a variety of places—soil, plants, fallen leaves, rotting wood, compost piles, grass, grain; if it's moist and dark, molds like it. When it gets warm, molds grow on plants that have died in the winter. As with the hives of stinging insects, try not to upset a mold source; doing so can disperse mold spores into the air.

There are many species of outdoor mold; only a few dozen are allergenic. Some molds, such as Cladosporium and Aspergillus, are regularly found both outdoors and in.

Outdoor landscape plants that look dirty are probably covered in mold spores. Plants that aren't thriving often become targets for insect pests, especially aphids, scale, and whitefly. Mold spores land, germinate, and proliferate on these plants. Remove any plants like this from your gardens.

If you suffer from mold allergy, typical fall activities like raking leaves, hiking, camping in the woods, and gardening might bring unpleasant symptoms.

To find out about elevated risk levels for mold in your locale, present or projected, visit pollen.com, the National Allergy Bureau website, or weather.com.

A Checklist for Traveling, Vacationing, and Being Away from Home

When you leave home and a familiar environment—for work or vacation, a short trip or extended stay, to a locale potentially less allergenic than home or more so—arm yourself with the information and, if needed, products to make your time away optimally pleasant and free of allergy disruption. Before traveling, check pollen counts and weather forecast for your destination; if you have flexibility, you might travel to avoid peak pollen season elsewhere.

WHAT TO BRING, DO, AND REQUEST:
- Pretreat. If your doctor has recommended oral/eye drop antihistamines and/or a prescription nasal spray, use them before you go so your next enclosed space—be it a room in a top hotel or an Airbnb rental—won't throw you.
- When flying, don't put allergy and asthma medications with your luggage, in case it's lost or stolen; include them with carry-ons.

- Bring refills, if needed. Finding allergy and asthma meds in other countries can be difficult and expensive. If you have enough, check the expiration dates.
- Moisturizing nasal saline gel, for longer flights, keeps nose moist.
- You may need a doctor's note to bring epinephrine auto-injectors through airport security.
- Bring an allergen-impermeable pillow casing, or at least a disposable pillow cover, to keep the "breathable space" when you sleep more allergen-free.
- Sunglasses block pollen, particularly when windy.
- Wash your hair nightly because pollen accumulates on skin and hair; you want to reduce its transfer to your boudoir, especially pillows and bedding. And no hair gel—it's a pollen trap.
- After you've been outside, irrigate eyelids gently with mild, tear-free shampoo.
- Exercise indoors, or at least avoid outdoors during early mornings, when pollen levels trend higher.
- You like the beach, a river, lake, other body of water, or the mountains? On the whole, pollen levels may be lower there. And high elevations (1,500+ meters) are associated with drier air, a less hospitable environment for house dust mites.
- When in cars, close windows and flip on the air conditioner (on the "no recirculate" setting).
- Reserve a non-smoking hotel room or—better, but less common—a "green"/allergy-friendly room. Wood, tile, or vinyl floors, if options, are all preferable to carpet.
- Request a non-smoking rental car, when possible.

Medication

To best manage symptoms of allergic rhinitis, what are the best medication choices?

For some, one medicine proves enough; others may need an array. As always with medication, there is the possibility of side effects; nasal decongestant spray especially may cause more trouble than the condition you're combating.

Over-the-counter (OTC) antihistamines may provide relief for itchy, watery eyes; sneezing; and runny nose, not for stuffiness/nasal congestion.

OTC nasal steroid spray may provide relief for both sets of symptoms.

OTC decongestant can decrease nasal/sinus congestion and stuffiness—however, as mentioned, taking a nasal decongestant for three or more days in a row may lead to rebound nasal congestion or rhinitis medicamentosa, which can feel worse than the original condition. (And frustrated patients, not realizing that their medication is worsening the problem, often continue to use the medication, making things worse still). Oral decongestant, both short- and long-acting, may cause unintended side effects such as increased heart rate and blood pressure, and insomnia.

Oral antihistamine may be combined with a decongestant.

Prescription medicine includes antihistamine nasal spray, which helps to reduce nasal inflammation and swelling, thus improving congestion, and tends to work fast (some in as little as fifteen to twenty minutes); a combination of an antihistamine with a corticosteroid nasal spray; and steroid nasal spray (which may take days to provide maximum relief). See also chapter 4, page 63, for more on medication.

OTC allergy eye medications may help to provide relief of red, itchy, watery eyes. It's best to avoid prolonged use of eye drops that also contain a decongestant. Prescription allergy medicine includes ocular antihistamine with mast cell–stabilizing eye drops, for itchy, watery eyes (mild side effects may include burning and/or stinging) and non-steroidal anti-inflammatory eye drops. See also chapter 4, page 63, for more on eye medication.

Treatment: Immunotherapy

For many people with seasonal allergy, allergen immunotherapy (also known as desensitization), which I talk about throughout the book but in more detail in chapter 10, can be effective in suppressing late-phase responses; in diminishing and stopping the progression of allergies to asthma, especially in children; and in providing long-term treatment of stinging insect allergy.

Chapter 6

Indoor Environment

▇

Maybe Americans don't live indoors entirely—but just about: On average, we spend 80 to 90 percent of our time inside our homes, workplaces, and other enclosed spaces. While our dwellings and other familiar indoor areas may feel like home, "strangers" lurk among us. One study found that more than half of homes contained at least six allergens; almost half had at least three allergens at levels exceeding the threshold for allergic sensitization and/or asthma. When you're in your home or office, are your nose, eyes, throat persistently irritated? House dust mites, pet dander, mold, and the like pose allergy risk inside your very home. We want to be extra careful about allergens in the home, especially for those with a family history of allergy and atopy.

The Peril Within

The hazards of our indoor spaces are numerous. For one, homes should probably be divided into two categories: those with pets and those without. All else being equal, the former group breeds a substantially heavier allergen load.

For another, unlike outdoor allergens, which tend to be seasonal or sporadic, indoor allergens are present year-round. We develop allergy, in part, based on the dose, proximity and duration of exposure. Because of the hours spent in a small series of enclosed spaces, for months and years, sensitization may eventually happen, followed by symptoms. And that number may go up, here and abroad: By 2030, three of every five people are projected to live in cities. Some researchers believe that in urban environments, airborne pollen grains attaching to circulating air pollutants (e.g., from vehicle emissions) can increase pollen's allergic potential, driving up allergic symptoms. A 2012 European study found that pollen counts in cities there were rising by an average of 3 percent a year, three times faster than the pollen count rise in rural areas.

Over the past decades, researchers have focused on the likely relationship between early exposure to indoor allergens and allergic sensitization, and asthma. Young children, from infants to toddlers to school-aged kids, may be at even greater risk since, on average, they spend more time indoors than do adults, and because early exposure to indoor allergens such as house dust mites, pet dander, mold, and cockroach and rodent allergen is associated with asthma (which may last into adulthood). The critical period for allergen sensitization appears to be the first two to three years of life. Sensitization to the major allergen in a given community may increase the likelihood of asthma in children from four to twenty times. A study of inner-city children showed a mind-boggling 94 percent of them with signs of allergic sensitization. With data like these, avoiding triggers is highly recommended, especially early in life, especially in cases where a family history exists.

Many of my patients have trouble with allergens they're exposed to outside the home—at work, at school or elsewhere—but hardly at all in their home; the latter is easier to remediate. In such cases, it can be harder to figure out the source of the problem and, when discovered, hard to change an environment not as much under their control.

This is all a largely new development. Our push for ever more energy-efficient, insulated homes is well-meaning (reduces greenhouse gases, lowers costs), and it's also intended, in a somewhat ironic twist, to protect us from the occasional perils of outdoors. Yet these new building designs often render indoor spaces warmer and more humid, paving the way for more house dust mites and mold (to name two), and reduces ventilation, facilitating an accumulation of allergens. (The new designs have helped spawn the term "sick building syndrome.") Open the window for better airflow—but are you inviting in mold, other plant allergens, and outdoor air pollution?

As referenced earlier, some studies seem to confirm the hygiene hypothesis: They show, for instance, that those who live on farms have lower rates of allergy than that of the general population. Is that all about being outdoors versus indoors? No, not exclusively. But the evidence is compelling.

Not all indoor spaces are equal. Differences that can have a direct effect on the type and level of allergens that build up indoors include:

- location of dwelling
- type of home (e.g., multistory apartment vs. private home)
- season (in those climate regions with three or four seasons, the period of summer/early fall means higher humidity, which means high mold levels, indoor and out)
- overall precipitation/dampness/humidity potential (which impacts mold growth)
- flooring type
- altitude (the higher your residence, the lower the level of house dust mites)

You can't rid your home of all traces of allergen, but the load can be reduced. The first keys are locating and isolating the allergen source.

> ## A Memorable Fact You Can't Un-Know (Sorry)
>
> ■
>
> That pillow you've used for two or more years, that now feels heavier? According to entomologists from Ohio State University, up to 10 percent of its weight is from droppings and dead dust mites (a significant portion of that increase is likely due to moisture). Wash pillows regularly in hot water; replace with new ones periodically.

Which Are the Indoor Allergens?

The majority of indoor allergens are protein compounds. They are found in parts of organisms (molds) and in the excretions and shed skin of insects, mites, and furred animals. They are carried along by particles of various shapes and sizes; they are found in indoor air; they can be inhaled.

If the allergen is small enough, it becomes easily airborne when the ambient air in the space is "disturbed." How long allergens remain airborne—thus, how much meaningful damage they may potentially cause—is dependent largely on their size/weight, somewhat less on their shape. When researchers attempt to determine the allergen load for an indoor space, they "dust sample" or "vacuum sample"—they vacuum settled dust on floors (including carpeting), furnishings, bedding, etc. (an inexact science, certainly). The dust is collected in a porous filtered container and processed in a laboratory. What have they found? After fifteen minutes of disturbance, most of the estimated house dust mite load has settled, while 10 to 20 percent of it remains airborne—the really, really small particles. The same is true for cockroach allergen. Because cat and dog allergen particles are generally smaller than 5 microns, the bulk remains airborne longer, making them more inhalable, potentially

Dust Never Sleeps: Quick Tips

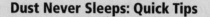

- Dust before you vacuum, so when you do vacuum, you catch particles that scattered.
- Dust top shelves first, then work your way down—again, so you capture, lower down or on the floor, what you scattered.
- Dust with a cloth that's damp, not dry.
- Use a vacuum equipped with a HEPA filter (or double-thickness bags).
- Thorough vacuuming once weekly beats not so thoroughly more often.
- The vacuum upholstery attachment is your friend. Use it on mattresses and padded furniture, favorite hangouts for house dust mites.

triggering immediate allergic symptoms. In short, whether an aeroallergen particle enters the lung air passage depends considerably on its size.

Other allergists and I have ranked the most common, intrusive indoor triggers, allergens likeliest to cause intermittent and/or persistent clinical allergy. This ranking is based not on definitive data (which does not yet exist) but on our perception, given what we treat on a regular basis:

1. house dust mites
2. cat dander
3. dog dander
4. mold spores
5. cockroach/mouse allergen
6. hamster, mouse, gerbil allergen

For those sensitized to indoor allergens, an environmental modification and remediation plan may include creating physical barriers, cleaning, and (as always) education.

There are really two basic aims for changing the indoor environment so that it poses a lesser allergy risk:

- Minimize the presence of particular allergens (source control).
- Minimize places where allergens can accumulate.

Home Allergen Remediation Strategies

What are the most common measures and techniques that you, or in some cases a hired expert, can take to reduce or eliminate indoor allergens?

Often one modification is not enough, and multiple strategies are recommended. Sometimes my first recommendations won't work. For instance, if a patient with a severe cat allergy won't give up her cat (I understand that) or a patient with a dust allergy won't remove her wall-to-wall carpet (harder to understand), we need another plan. Many allergy sufferers have multiple triggers, so a multipronged approach is best.

Surfaces both hard and soft must be considered. Certain areas of the home are particularly troublesome.

a. Physical measures. Modification efforts include adding barriers such as allergen-impermeable fabric bedding covers (pillow, box spring, mattress, duvet, furniture covers); airtight, zippered plastic covers; and woven fabrics whose openings should be small enough to prevent passage of house dust mite allergen but large enough still to permit good airflow; adding easy-to-clean blinds that are wiped weekly with a damp cloth, and washable shades rather than non-washable drapes and blinds; laundering bedding and clothing frequently in 130°F (55 to 60°C) water.

b. Soft surface measures. Avoid carpets and rugs—but consider washable rugs. Porous/stuffed toys that may be rich reservoirs for dust mites should be placed in a freezer bag for twenty-four hours to kill the allergen. (But for this to be effective, you'll want to run the toys in the dryer to remove remaining dust particles, and repeat the whole process at least weekly.) Opt for furniture and furnishings less likely to attract or harbor allergen, such as washable furnishings, leather, metal, plastic, etc.

c. *Hard surface measures.* Preferred flooring: wood, tile, polished floors, and linoleum rather than carpets. For smooth flooring, vacuuming (with a HEPA-filter vacuum) and damp mopping is effective. Using disinfecting/moist wipes, wet vacuuming, and anti-mildew measures that include the use of EPA-registered products will help to prevent and manage mold and mildew growth. Beginning around 2009, several OTC consumer-branded products such as anti-allergen, mold-control solutions and sprays came onto the market to help remove indoor allergens from surfaces. (Data provided by manufacturers often vary in their allergy-fighting capability.)

d. *Clothing and fabrics.* Hot-cycle (130°F, or 55°C to 60°C) washing kills dust mites.

e. *Mechanical devices.* HEPA air filters appear to be beneficial in reducing airborne pet dander. High-efficiency whole house filtration, with portable HEPA air purifiers, may provide some benefit. For those with dust mite and/or mold allergy, humidifiers and vaporizers should probably not be used in the bedroom. Ideally, indoor humidity will be kept below 50 percent. Steam-cleaning can kill mites in carpets.

f. *Building and engineering controls.* Superior ventilation, basement fans, mold-resistant materials and flooring, central AC, and central heating all help to reduce allergen load. Home inspection (especially searching out roof leaks) by a contractor can be helpful, as is maintenance of these systems.

RODENT

With one very big exception, allergy to rodents is more likely a problem for those who work with mice and rats in labs. Still, guinea pigs, hamsters, and gerbils are common house pets, and rodent allergen may be present in the home without one's awareness, since mice and rats remain largely hidden. Because mouse allergen is transported on small, often airborne particles, it can make its way into homes with no mouse infestation.

Which brings me to that very big exception: Inner-city, multifamily homes virtually all have mouse allergen. In suburban homes, the rate is approximately 50 to 75 percent. The key difference is not the incidence in inner-city homes but the extent: It may be a hundred to a thousand times greater than what's detected in suburban homes. Worse, the level in inner-city schools often exceeds that in nearby homes. Asthma is found at epidemic levels in the inner city; a risk factor for asthma is sensitization to rodent allergen, and exposure to rats and mice correlates with an increase in asthma symptoms.

To reduce rodent infestation, avoidance isn't enough. Integrated pest management—targeted application of low-toxicity pesticides, plugging access to indoor areas (cracks and crevices with copper mesh, caulk sealant, etc.), placing snap traps, preventing access to food—is generally required. You must be strenuously, persistently committed to maintaining the newly clean areas.

Over time, mice can develop resistance to rodenticides.

Ultrasonic devices have been used to deter mice from entering homes, but evidence of their effectiveness remains unpersuasive.

COCKROACH

Cockroaches are very mobile, so they can spread their allergen widely and sometimes elusively—in kitchens (behind appliances, in hard-to-reach crevices) and in bedding. The two species that Americans contend with most: the American cockroach, or water bug, the largest species of common cockroach and one that tends to live outdoors or in sewers, and may be the dominant indoor species in tropical areas; and the German cockroach, the most common variety in the northeastern United States. Cockroach droppings, body parts, and saliva contain allergens. Researchers can detect cockroach allergen during or after vacuum cleanings. As with rodent infestation, the allergen is more detectable in inner-city dwellings, particularly in high-rise buildings. Studies have shown an association between the presence and quantity of these allergens with kids' hospitalization for asthma.

Cockroaches flourish in environments that are damp and warm or hot, particularly where sources of food and water are available; not surprisingly, the bathroom and kitchen tend to harbor the greatest population of roaches. Place sticky traps near food or water sources to assess infestation and see if the problem is contained. Ground zero for cockroach allergen? The kitchen floor, particularly in urban high-rises.

Cockroach allergen may also be detected in meaningful concentration in the bedroom (in crevices), on the living room floor, and in upholstery.

When cleaning, start with the least toxic method of roach control. Seek the advice of a licensed exterminator for the most effective, safe approach.

- Repair leaks immediately.
- Plug holes to the house from outside, plus holes in cabinets, cupboards, and walls.
- Don't leave food out. Eliminate crumbs. Keep food out of other rooms. Store food in sealed containers.

INDOOR AIR POLLUTION

How do you improve indoor air quality? Remove what's bad. Control the source of any pollution, and allow for superior ventilation.

- Minimize use of chemicals and products known for their power-ful odor and/or which are irritants, such as cleaning products, air freshener, essential oils with diffusers, hair spray, insect spray, paint (fumes), and smoke.
- Try environment-friendly products that are easily found in stores such as Whole Foods.
- Cap humidity at 30 to 50 percent. An inexpensive hygrometer will monitor humidity.
- Air-conditioning minimizes outdoor pollen and/or molds.
- Reduce or eliminate airborne contaminants or odors by install-ing an exhaust fan near the source, vented to outdoors.
- If you use a fireplace or fuel-burning appliance, good ventilation is vital.
- Open windows.

Flowers to the Rescue

A proper mix of plants is good for us: A study in Finland found that a yard where a diverse blend of "uncommon, native flower plants" grew was associated with healthy immune system functioning of those who lived there. Think about it: If your outdoor environment has that kind of effect, your indoor one is likely even more impactful. To improve in-door air, keep out the bad—and our national space agency has contrib-uted to the effort. The well-publicized NASA Clean Air Study, published in 1989, includes a list of houseplants that help to filter indoor air of common toxic chemicals such as benzene, formaldehyde, trichloroeth-ylene, xylene, toluene, and ammonia. You can help clean indoor air in a home or office by having one 10- to 12-inch potted plant for every 100 square feet of space.

Note: Indoor plants will clean air only if they're strong and healthy. Sickly plants won't do it, and might even cause new problems.

THE BEST HOUSEPLANTS TO TRY

Common names vary, so verify plants by their botanical names.

- Aloe vera
- Areca palm
- Bamboo palm or reed palm
- Boston fern
- Chinese evergreen
- Corn cane or mass cane
- Cornstalk dracaena
- Dwarf/pygmy date palm
- Elephant ear philodendron
- English ivy
- Gerbera daisy or Barberton daisy
- Golden pothos or devil's ivy
- Heartleaf philodendron
- Janet Craig dracaena
- Kimberly queen fern
- Lady palm (10+ varieties)
- Marginata or dragon tree
- Moth orchid
- Mum
- Peace lily
- Philodendron
- Pot mum or florist's chrysanthemum
- Red-edged dracaena
- Rubber plant
- Schefflera
- Snake plant or mother-in-law's tongue
- Spider plant
- Warneck dracaena
- Weeping fig

A few cautions:

- Some of these plants may be harmful if children or pets put them in their mouth. For more information on plant safety, check out aspca.org/pet-care/animal-poison-control/toxic-and-non-toxic-plants.
- The ficus (including the rubber tree) is a big producer of VOCs (volatile organic compounds) and will not improve indoor air quality.
- Some of these plants, such as the spider plant, produce considerable male flowers and shed allergenic pollen indoors.
- Ferns are tricky to grow inside; when they do thrive, they produce spores, which are allergenic.

House Dust Mites (HDM)

We shed about one-fifth of an ounce of dead skin each week. This organic matter is ingested by microscopic insects called house dust mites, which are so prevalent in homes that the scientific community awarded them their own acronym, HDM. They're found the world over, and at least thirteen species of mite have been identified in house dust.

A link between HDMs and asthmatic symptoms was first suggested in 1921; in the 1960s, HDMs were called out as a prime cause. When the allergen exceeds a certain level, it can provoke asthma symptoms in sensitive individuals.

Of the top indoor allergens, HDMs are the ones to which we most commonly develop sensitization. Even the cleanest home has them. One survey found dust mite allergen in 85 percent of the homes surveyed. Dust mites are resilient and may take months to die, and it may take even longer for their allergens to significantly decrease, particularly from such prime hosts as bedding, mattresses, and carpeting.

Some good news, though: They have very particular needs for growing. Eliminate those sources, and mites can be reduced fairly easily. En-

Outside In

■

It's nice to have a Christmas tree in your living room to make the holidays more festive—but a few things for the allergic to consider:

- Many people have worsening asthma and allergy symptoms when they bring a pine tree indoors. The pine itself is rarely the problem. It's usually the mold on the branches and needles (which can occur on both real and artificial trees).
- Before bringing your tree indoors, thoroughly shake it out (the place where you buy it may have precisely such a machine), then set it outside to dry in a covered area for a few days. *Then* bring it indoors.
- Before showering the tree with artificial snow or flocking, remember that inhaling the spray may irritate the lungs and potentially trigger asthma symptoms.
- The fragrance of a Christmas tree may trigger a reaction. This is one time where a fake may beat the real thing.
- If you go the artificial tree route, dust it off before displaying it each year. Same for decorations that have been stored for almost a year.
- Holiday decorations made of metal, glass, and plastic keep relatively dust-free; those made of soft fabric, not so much.
- Given all the new, foreign substances you're about to bring into your home, under one roof, in a contained space, be proactive: Premedicate with necessary OTC and prescribed medications before symptoms can kick into gear.

vironmental factors—temperature, humidity, season—influence the impact of HDMs. They can't survive in humidity below 40 to 50 percent. Mites flourish in warm, humid weather, and year-round in the mid/southern Atlantic coastal areas and Gulf coastal regions. In a 2011 compilation by Quest Diagnostics of the worst big American cities for allergies, the city with the lowest rate of sensitization to HDMs was Denver. Given the altitude of the Mile High City, thus the drier air, it's an inhospitable area for dust mites.

WAYS TO REDUCE DUST MITE EXPOSURE

Turn on that air conditioner or dehumidifier: Reduces humidity, ergo dust mites. Maintain relative humidity below 50 percent. In dry climates, this is easily accomplished by regularly opening windows; in humid climates, by using air-conditioning. While dehumidifiers may also help, they do not filter air the way air conditioners do. If you have dry nasal passages, use saline nasal gel spray or other directed remedies before bed rather than humidifying the entire bedroom.

Invest in a HEPA vacuum: Regularly vacuum using a HEPA filter or double-layered microfilter bag.

Remove/clean the favored nests of HDMs: House dust mites are found abundantly in bedding—pillows, mattresses, box springs, curtains, blankets, duvets, etc.—plus soft furniture and furnishings, couches and sofas, carpets and rugs, and other woven materials. Both dry heat and commercial steam treatments can eradicate dust mites. Wash sheets, pillowcases, mattress pads, and blankets weekly. I recommend hot water with detergent, and an electric clothes dryer on the hot setting. Note that it's the high temperature, not the detergent, that kills dust mites. Dust mite–impermeable bedding covers may help but are not sufficient by themselves.

Some helpful points (not all of which are easy or aesthetically pleasing):

- Bedrooms are (ideally) carpet-free. Upholstered furniture anywhere in the home is not recommended.
- Easy-to-wipe window coverings or blinds are better than drapes.
- A damp rag or mop is better for removing dust.
- If choosing woven fabrics, ask about pore size of roughly 6 mi-

crons, small enough to block the passage of immature and adult live dust mites as well as cat allergen, but large enough for sufficient airflow.

* Encase pillows (remove decorative ones) and mattresses in allergen-impermeable covers.
* Vacuum mattress, pillows, and the base of the bed.
* Synthetic bedding is preferable to feather or wool, and handles frequent washing in hot water.

Studies of how to kill dust mites or to denature allergens with chemicals (active ingredients: benzyl benzoate, tannic acid), few of which have been marketed in the United States, have reported only modest success so far.

Room by Room

Can home cleaning provide an anti-allergic effect in asthma patients? The evidence suggests yes, particularly if the cleanup is just one of several steps. I believe it's worth it. Here are some steps to take, going around the house.

WHOLE HOME

For patients with allergic respiratory disease, I may—depending on the circumstances—recommend air filtration as one of several environmen-

Lazy Pays

■

A study from Kingston University in the United Kingdom found that beds left unmade, so that sheets were exposed to the air, left them drier, significantly reducing their dust mite content.

tal modification efforts, particularly if they are pet-allergic and cannot realistically part with their animal. As a stand-alone effort, though, it's probably not enough. For home modification to be more effective, certain major allergen reservoirs, such as carpeting, old furniture and other dust collectors, may need to be removed. Still, using a dehumidifier throughout the house, or in areas that need it, reduces dampness. Make sure to clean the dehumidifier weekly.

Better flooring can help to reduce allergen load home-wide. Limit the presence of carpets. No carpet dust means far smaller volume of dust mites and other allergens that reside there. Remove moldy or water-damaged carpeting. Alternatively, hard surfaces are easily cleaned with a dust mop and leave no asylum for allergens to hide. Surfaces to consider include hardwood, cork (suberin, its natural antimicrobial, reduces mold, mildew, and bacteria growth), bamboo (water-resistant, and less likely than hardwood to retain moisture), ceramic tile, stone, concrete, linoleum, laminate, vinyl, and porcelain.

Examine the house foundation, windows, and any stairwells for leaks or water damage. Repair the source.

BEDROOM

The number one allergy hotspot is the bedroom. It's where we spend approximately one-third of each day, magnifying the lurking allergen load since we're exposed to it for so many hours. While sleeping, our breath and perspiration create humidity. The area around the bed is a "microenvironment" where indoor allergens may flourish—it's warm and somewhat humid. It can take just four months for mattresses and box springs not "protected" to reach peak levels, so using barriers such as allergen-impermeable covers may reduce HDM allergen compared to bedding without encasings. Pillows, blankets, comforters, and duvets should be regularly washed in hot water.

Carpeting and Upholstered Furnishing: Aside from the bed, major reservoirs of indoor allergen are carpet and upholstered furnishing, which can harbor dust mites in high humidity. The greatest concentration of indoor dust mites is in bedding and flooring (along with living room upholstery). To control them, lowering humidity may be more effective than surface carpet treatments, whose impact may only be short-lived, perhaps because HDM allergen increases the lower and deeper you get in the carpet. While dry vacuum-cleaning picks up excess dust, wet vacuum-cleaning may be two to three times more effective, according to one study. Steam that's superheated can also kill mites in carpets.

If possible, ditch upholstered furnishings (sofas, chairs) for wood-, metal-, leather-, or plastic-based furniture.

Closets: High indoor humidity can cause mold to grow on many items, including clothing. Keep indoor humidity between 30 and 50 percent. If it's not humid outside, open windows or doors to allow in fresh air.

Corners: Moisture from a roof leak may seep into the wall, causing paint to buckle and peel. Don't paint over wet/moldy walls.

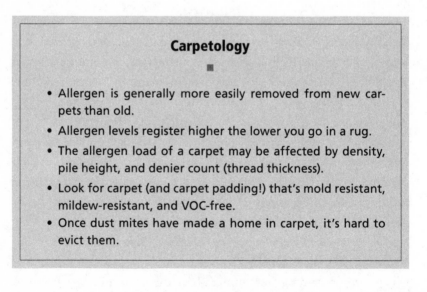

Carpetology

- Allergen is generally more easily removed from new carpets than old.
- Allergen levels register higher the lower you go in a rug.
- The allergen load of a carpet may be affected by density, pile height, and denier count (thread thickness).
- Look for carpet (and carpet padding!) that's mold resistant, mildew-resistant, and VOC-free.
- Once dust mites have made a home in carpet, it's hard to evict them.

LIVING ROOM

Walls: Hidden leaks may cause wet spots on walls, leading to mold growth behind walls. A professional can find the source and fix the problem. If you have wallpaper, consider replacing it with tile, or using enamel paint that's mold-resistant.

Windows: Condensation can be a sign of high indoor humidity, which has many possible causes and should be investigated.

Fireplace: Because gases and smoke can worsen respiratory allergy symptoms, avoid wood-burning stoves or fireplaces, where possible. Natural-gas fireplaces are generally fine.

KITCHEN

Stove: Use a stove's exhaust hood (vented to the outdoors) to draw out heat, moisture, and other contaminants; not all stove hoods do this.

Refrigerator: Moisture breeds mold, so minimize buildup by emptying the drip pan and keeping rubber door seals clean. Beware mystery foods in the back of the fridge that become gardens of mold.

Sink: Keep it free of dirty dishes, and scrubbed (along with faucets).

Cabinets and Counters: A detergent-water mix keeps them clean. Use sealed containers to store food. Leaking pipes under the sink can lead to mold growth in walls or cabinets. Professional plumbing services may be required.

BATHROOM

Shower, bathtub: Run the exhaust fan (if there is one) or open the window when showering to avoid buildup of excessive moisture. (For bathrooms with no window or fan, be vigilant to keep mold growth at bay.) Afterward, wipe tub and surrounding area dry. If mold develops around faucets, shower, and/or tub, use an EPA-registered mildew cleaner or a natural alternative product (ensure proper ventilation and safety measures are in place). Don't wait for bathmats and shower curtains to turn moldy before investing in new ones.

Toilet and sink: Mold often develops around fixtures; check and scrub regularly. Beware leaks.

BASEMENT

A dehumidifier helps to prevent mold growth. Clean it regularly, per manufacturer instructions.

Use plastic storage bins to store clothes and other such items.

LAUNDRY ROOM

Clothes dryer: It should be vented to the outdoors.

Laundry: Bedding is optimally washed in water 130°F (155°C) or hotter. Tumble dry clothes in a hot dryer.

FRONT DOOR

Double up on welcome mats: About 85 percent of the contaminants in your home lurk within three to four steps of your exterior door(s). Having two doormats—one just outside, one inside—at every exit point can make a difference. Shake them out every few days.

OUTSIDE

Roof: A professional should evaluate wet spots or water stains.

Yard: Gutters should be long enough to draw rainwater at least 5 feet away from the foundation. Water pooling around the foundation can lead to indoor moisture problems. The ground near a house should be sloped away from it.

Pets/Animals

Pet ownership is the strongest predictor of a home's allergen load. Given the roughly 100 million pets in US homes, equally divided between cats and dogs, that's a lot of allergen. Cat and dog allergen register in air samples from every home that's got pets—and in many without, too, likely because of the allergen's portability and stickiness on clothing. The levels detected in homes without pets are not insignificant: They are often high enough to correlate to an increased risk of sensitization. Cat allergen is particularly ubiquitous, with marked levels detectable— as anyone who knows cats would expect—in living room upholstery and on beds.

Animal allergen is spread largely via scales shed from the animal's skin—the dander—that then sticks to surfaces; asthma and allergy can also be triggered by the animal's urine, feces, saliva, and hair. Dog and cat allergen particles are small, thus often airborne, unlike house dust mites, whose structure and larger size make them more likely to settle on flooring.

The most effective way to deal with pet allergen is to get rid of the animal. Of course, I get that that's not a practical solution for most pet owners. Thorough cleaning and dust removal can help reduce the allergen load.

And for those who *really* don't like the idea of eliminating the pet as a way to be free (or freer) of allergy, how about this interesting study: Sleeping on animal fur during infancy has been shown to lower asthma risk.

CAT

Cat allergen (Fel d 1) is sticky and small, about one-tenth the size of dust mite allergen, and often carried on clothing—and it's stubborn. One researcher found that air cleaning is not generally efficient to reduce exposure; bathing and keeping the pet from the bedroom weren't much

---

Dogs 1, Cats 0

■

Cat allergy is more prevalent than dog allergy not because of dander or fur but likely the relative petiteness of cat protein, hosted in cat fur and skin: It is light enough to remain airborne for hours. The particle size enables it to be breathed deep into the lungs.

---

help, either. For allergen levels in carpets to return to those of homes without cats can take up to twenty weeks; for mattresses, five years! Simply put, cat allergen cannot be totally removed. It is most prevalent in the bed, bedding, and floor, and the living room/family room floor and upholstery. It adheres to soft furnishings, including couches, chairs, chaises, and mattresses, as well as in carpet dust.

One study showed that high-efficiency filtration in a central forced air system eliminated more than half of airborne cat allergen. Aggressive cleaning is required. Carpet accumulates cat allergen at a rate roughly one hundred times that of a floor that's smooth and polished.

Washing cats less than weekly is unlikely to improve things much. Some studies show that airborne cat allergen returns to pre-bath levels in as little as one to three days. Since cats are generally not fans of bathing, frequent cat-washing is much easier said than done.

Litter boxes may contain some of the highest amounts of cat allergen, due to concentration of allergen found in the cat's anal glands. Even when the box is removed from the room, evidence of the allergen is noticeable to susceptible, sensitive visitors (as yours truly can attest).

DOG

In homes with a dog, carpet dust is where dog allergen (Can f 1) is predominantly found (aside from on the dog itself).

Frequent dog-washing may significantly reduce the presence of aller-

---

Myth: There are non-allergenic breeds of dog (bichon frise, Maltese, poodle, miniature schnauzer) and cat (e.g., Siberian, Siamese, Sphynx).

■

The word *hypoallergenic* means "less likely to cause allergy" or "slightly allergenic"—but colloquially it has come to mean non-allergenic. With dogs and cats, there is no such beast. Indeed, there's no convincing evidence that one breed is less or more allergenic than any other. No relationship has yet been proved between the length of pet hair and its allergen content. (After all, the allergen is not in the fur but in the animal's saliva, dander, and urine.) The allergen is a protein that all dogs and cats carry, so there is no allergy-free breed.

However, each animal *is* different—some cat breeds manufacture less of the allergy-triggering protein Fel d I—and you may do better with one breed than another. Some people *do* feel better around a breed that has shorter hair or sheds less. There is anecdotal evidence that allergy sufferers may do better with a dog that keeps its coat. And if you're going to bathe your animal regularly, it makes sense to consider his or her potential disposition in the bath.

---

gen; the level of airborne allergen noticeably decreases. Unfortunately, maintaining that reduction requires twice-a-week washings, an impractical burden for many dog owners. HEPA air cleaning can meaningfully reduce airborne dog allergen.

Removing carpets and other allergen reservoirs can provide some reduction. Isolating the pet in a separate area of the home may provide benefit—but given your feeling for your dog, this might not be an option.

OTHER PETS

A growing number of exotic animals, including reptiles, birds, insects, rodents, ferrets, and monkeys, are kept as pets, and allergic responses to these animals are reported. Avian (bird) proteins are found not only in homes with birds (often in house dust), but also in homes with feather comforters, quilts, duvets, down-filled jackets, and pillows. Feathers can contain dander, and their shape and structure may influence the amount of mite allergen. For years, the conventional wisdom was that "allergic kids" ought to avoid feather pillows. But a recent study suggests that feather pillows do not accumulate dust mites, at least as measured over the course of three months.

Exposure to ferrets, which are sometimes kept as pets, has been reported in the literature to be a potential allergen, thus can trigger asthma in sensitive individuals. Hamster and gerbil allergy are also not uncommon.

THE ANIMAL ALLERGEN LOAD-DOWN

Home modifications to help reduce animal allergen:

- Find a new home for your pet.
- Keep your pet outside.
- Choose a low-dander pet rather than a furry or feathered friend.

. . . and if none of that works?

- Make the bedroom off-limits.
- Try to make furniture off-limits. (Good luck with that.)
- Get zippered plastic cases for pillows and mattresses. (You can purchase covers of varying qualities of comfortable fabrics.)
- Get rid of carpet.
- Clean frequently with a vacuum affixed with a HEPA filter or double-layered microfilter bag.

Mold

If you've experienced substantial flooding and are concerned about mold in your home, get help from an experienced, insured specialist in cleaning and restoration, to determine appropriate steps to take to mitigate any mold problem.

There's evidence linking indoor exposure to mold with upper respiratory tract symptoms, cough, and wheeze in people who are otherwise healthy. Higher rates of mold in the home are associated with higher rates of asthma (though we can't say for sure that indoor mold alone causes childhood asthma). Mold does not have to be of the ugly, smelly "black mold" variety to cause a problem. That doesn't mean we can ignore mold until it's obvious—and even then it might not be, since it often grows in relative secrecy, such as in air ducts and cavities behind walls.

Handheld meters measure moisture levels in various materials, and may help to track down areas of biologic growth; if you're just "eyeballing" a potential problem around the home, you may miss it. Your home could have a significant mold problem that cannot be smelled, either. You can't see an individual mold without a microscope, but you can observe it when it has colonized, as on an old slice of bread or a bathroom ceiling. Mold allergy symptoms are the same as those for allergies to other airborne particles.

A huge majority of dust samples taken from US homes—over 95 percent—have detectable levels of the mold Alternaria. In the South and West (at lower altitudes), outdoor molds can be found year-round; in the North, mold counts are elevated during late summer and early fall. (For most of the United States, mold counts peak in early fall and in May.) There is no consistent federal limit for acceptable levels of mold spores in any indoor environment, despite the fact that the presence of mold in your home increases your children's risk of developing asthma. While mold is ever present, its level varies dramatically with a number of factors: urban dwellings, perceived or observed moisture problems, presence of pets, geographic effects, presence of humidifier, and age of home.

Mold spores need moisture to grow; they prefer relative humidity of 65 percent or more, temperature between 50°F and 90°F (10°C and 32°C), and organic or synthetic matter for food.

Some factors that promote indoor mold spore growth include the use of humidifiers, and stored organic materials and/or soil. Mold spores are found in higher amounts in homes with wall-to-wall carpets. Water-soaked carpets/rugs and basement floor surfaces can be a frequent source of mold and mildew. Other areas typically associated with mold growth include bathroom surfaces, shower stalls and curtains, kitchen sinks, food storage areas, wall coverings, dirty and soiled upholstery, and garbage containers. Contaminated air ducts and filters can harbor molds.

The initial inspection for indoor mold includes examination for musty odors and visible mold on surfaces. Visible mold can be remediated without further testing.

To prevent mold growth, the structure and furnishings should be kept as dry as possible. Aside from keeping surfaces and structures dry, locate and eliminate, or at least reduce, moisture sources. Adequately ventilate water-prone areas, such as bathrooms and laundry areas. Remove standing water. Avoid rugs/carpets on top of cement flooring.

Bring down humidity by increasing ventilation, covering cold surfaces such as water pipes with insulation, and raising air temperature.

Another inexpensive but effective means of removing surface mold is to scrub contaminated nonporous hard surfaces with detergent and water, then dry the area completely. You may use disinfectant products registered with the EPA to manage mold and mildew, such as branded disinfectant sprays, disinfecting wipes, and mold and mildew removers, some of which contain bleach. Ventilate the area adequately.

Other ways to address the mold problem include using mold- and mildew-resistant materials, paints, and coatings, and removing vegetation and excessive numbers of indoor plants.

Any contaminated areas in which mold has embedded itself, such as a porous wall, floor, carpet, or upholstered area, need to be removed or replaced. If professional remediation is required, a certified industrial hygienist is preferred.

Should You Be Scared of "Black Mold"?

■

"Black mold" or "toxic mold" is less commonly found in the home than many other indoor molds. It often grows after damage from flooding, water leaks, and in other conditions of high humidity. In general, molds are neither toxic nor poisonous. Certain molds can be toxigenic: They produce toxins, notably mycotoxins, but the particular hazards that these molds present are reportedly similar to those of other common household molds. According to most of the literature, it's rare to hear of toxigenic, in-home molds causing unusual health conditions. Still, opportunists may claim that exposure to "toxic mold" is the cause for many symptoms. There's a link between indoor molds and a variety of respiratory symptoms, including cough, wheezing, and symptoms of allergic asthma. The CDC's guidelines recommend mold prevention and remediation efforts, regardless of the mold species (including *Stachybotrys chartarum*, the mold often known as black mold).

TIPS TO REDUCE MOLD EXPOSURE

- Use a dehumidifier or air conditioner to reduce humidity. When you turn on the AC, vacate the room briefly, as mold spores may disperse.
- Make regular rounds of your faucets, pipes, and ductwork to catch water buildup early.
- Avoid using carpet or wallpaper, particularly in areas that tend to dampness (e.g., basement, ground floor).
- Kitchen, bathrooms, and other damp regions should have exhaust fans. Clothes dryers should be vented to the outside.
- Don't let decaying debris build up on the roof, in gutters, or in the yard. If you're allergic to mold, let someone else rake, mow, and work with mulch.

- If you come across mold, use a solution of 1 part chlorine to 10 parts water to eliminate it.
- Often the mold problem is outside—but right near the home. If a tree that needs good light is planted in the shade, it will often become buggy, then soon after be covered with sooty mold. (It will look dirty.) Water from irrigation sprinklers hitting the side of the house can cause mold issues. And overwatered lawns often get heavy with mold. Bark mulch, which often sits right beside the house, may harbor large amounts of mold.

Medication

See Medication in chapter 5 (page 109), for information on medicines to relieve symptoms of year-round allergy.

Chapter 7

Skin Allergies

Skin allergies are generally not common in children. Many of those who come to my office with skin conditions are in their twenties to forties. Often they're suffering from allergic contact dermatitis, and the triggering substances are the yet-to-be-identified elements of their daily habits and interactions: makeup; fragrances; metal in their jewelry, accessories, and phone; products in their homes (especially in the kitchen or bathroom) and at work; and rubber. I see more of these allergies than when I started my practice twenty years ago. I also see three times as many hives cases as I did.

Why the increase and change in type? The "easier" stuff has fallen away. Thanks to the greater availability of OTC medications like Benadryl, Claritin, and Allegra, there is more self-medication. For treatment of nonelusive conditions, many patients bypass doctors in favor of the convenience, speed, and reasonable expense of a walk-in urgent care clinic. If there's a sense that the situation can be "fixed" with a cream or some other medication, patients often go there. I'd estimate the volume of more complex cases in my offices has tripled compared to a decade ago. While I start patients on medication right away to relieve itching, it takes a thorough investigation to get at the root of the problem. And because it's often not a root but *roots*—a condition that's "multifactorial"—what presents clearly (e.g., hives) is often not so simple to solve. An urgent care clinic may be the best option if you have *only* hives and your interaction with the trigger was fleeting enough that the condition resolves. But what if the cause of the hives requires more investigative work? What if the contact was not the sole reason for the outbreak on the skin, or other symptoms? The complexity is understood best when seen as a pie chart:

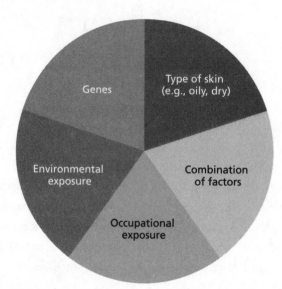

When dealing with skin conditions, it's important to ask questions like:

How does the condition of the skin affect the likelihood of a reaction? (Dry, abraded, or otherwise unhealthy skin that lacks an intact barrier is more vulnerable than healthy, intact skin.)

What clues does the skin's appearance provide about underlying causes? Is it the original rash or has the appearance changed from so much scratching? Is it itchy or not? Is the affected area raised or flat?

Itching to Know

■

An itch (medical term: *pruritus*) is the uncomfortable sensation of needing to scratch; in various skin and other conditions, an itch is, in part, usually sparked by the immune system's release of histamine (known as the "itch chemical").

Non-allergic conditions such as dry skin can cause itching. Other possible causes include adverse effects to medication, thyroid conditions, and kidney or liver disease. Less commonly, a hematology evaluation may help to uncover possible underlying medical conditions where there is generalized itching after your skin condition or rash is evaluated.

Ironically—or maybe not—another cause of itching is . . . scratching.

Could the skin condition be the result of contact with something solid, liquid, or airborne, something ingested or touched?

Is the affected area only where it touched the allergen or irritant, or has it spread beyond that, the result of an intense immune/inflammation response?

What did the patient apply to the affected area? (The suspected substance may have many components, including the active ingredient, preservatives, and fragrances. For example, I've had multiple patients turn out to be allergic to topical steroid cream, and while for some the allergen was the preservative used in the cream, for others it was the steroid component; and there are various classes of steroids, so certain patients may tolerate some but not others.)

Which tests might help to solve the mystery?

Yes, Non-Medication Strategies Really *Do* Help

■

Recently, I had a consultation with Julie, a thirty-five-year-old hairstylist. She'd just had another bout of intermittent skin rash, which covered her arms, torso, and neck. I asked her a bunch of basic questions, then queried her a little more about her work and home situation. She had broken up with her boyfriend several weeks before her itchy, unbearable rash kicked into gear. After our visit, she improved initially on non-sedating antihistamines that seemed to control her skin-related distress. But I also had her take a standard patient questionnaire about her perceived level of anxiety; she scored very high. She was not all better: Her emotional highs and lows seemed to impact her symptoms. I looked into, and soon excluded, the possibility that one or more of the products and hair treatments at her salon contained chemicals that triggered her rash. Julie also sought the advice of a therapist, and started on a number of self-help interventions to deal with her recent heightened emotions. These interventions included daily exercise, yoga, and other non-medication approaches such as mindfulness training and positive imagery. Before long, her daily rash and severe itchiness were occurring with less frequency. She was considerably better, and not just on her skin (though that was likely helped by topical skin moisturizers that hydrate the skin—oils, petrolatum and emollient). Some research states that recent stressful events are often associated with the onset of dermatitis and/or hives.

After several months, Julie's chronic hives had become so much less uncomfortable that for periods she was able to reduce her reliance on antihistamines; the cycle of less scratching and less stress fed on each other, in a good way.

The mind-body connection is increasingly respected as a factor in stress-induced conditions.

Substances That Contain Ingredients That Can Cause Skin Allergy

■

- cleansers
- deodorants
- dyes
- excipients (inactive ingredients or fillers)
- fragrances
- glues
- metals
- preservatives
- sunscreens

Eczema

Eczema runs the gamut from mild to moderate to severe.

While the root causes of eczema are complex and not entirely understood—it's believed to be caused by a mix of factors including genetics, environment, immune system abnormalities, and activities causing the skin to be more sensitive—the resulting condition is relatively simple: Because the skin barrier is failing at some of its key responsibilities (letting moisture out, and germs and irritants in), allergens penetrate more easily, allowing infectious organisms such as staph bacteria to invade.

Male Skin vs. Female Skin

■

Male skin tends to be oilier and reddens more easily than female skin; the pores are larger and the skin is more vulnerable to impurities and acne; that might factor into my decision to prescribe a topical cream or gel, given the oil content of certain medications. Also, shaving removes the top layer of skin, rendering the skin sensitive to outside invaders, such as irritants and skin allergens.

The cycle of itch and scratch is under way, and more areas of the skin become vulnerable to the cells that ignite the response. This may culminate in more widespread, persistent disease.

How does one know if it's atopic eczema or extra-dry skin? Diagnosing atopic eczema (aka atopic dermatitis) involves examining the skin, as well as taking a history of the patient and her family. The majority of those who suffer from the condition have a family history of allergy— not necessarily eczema but hay fever or asthma—as well. (The prevalence in one family of all three conditions is dubbed "atopic triad.") Roughly four in five children with eczema develop hay fever and/or asthma; one-third to nearly two-thirds of kids and young people who suffer from eczema also have food allergy.

Eczema's area of concentration can change. Sometimes it's located around the hand or foot, sometimes around the mouth, and its appearance and treatment can also differ. Various substances and environments make eczema flare. It's a condition where the itch almost always precedes the rash; it's an itch that rashes, which differentiates it from other conditions that are rashes that itch (like psoriasis), where the lesions are present before the overt skin symptoms such as itch become a concern.

Some common eczema triggers:

- hormones (flare-ups occur due to hormonal changes, particularly in women)
- irritants (including bubble bath, shampoos, and soaps; detergents, dishwashing liquid, disinfectants, and other cleaning products; fragranced chemicals, perfumes, and skin care products; rough fabric; juice from fresh fruits; vegetables, nuts, and even animal sources)
- allergens (including house dust mite, pet dander, pollen, mold, and fabric dye)
- microbes (including bacteria such as staph, viruses, fungi)
- foods (including dairy products, eggs, nuts, wheat, seeds, soy products)

- extremes in temperature and humidity, including perspiration from exercise
- stress
- sun (a trigger for some, a treatment for others)

Eczema cannot be cured. However, its severity may be reduced significantly by taking some of these measures . . .

- Avoid triggers as much as possible.
- Use clothing and blankets made of white cotton rather than wool and other fabric that can irritate the skin.
- Maintain indoor moisture level of less than 50 percent. An inexpensive hygrometer helps to monitor the range. Humid air, good; dry air, bad.
- Short, tepid showers are recommended. Apply a cream moisturizer when just out of the shower; when the body is moist, absorption increases. It's particularly important to hydrate the skin well during the winter.
- Use less rubbing force while bathing and drying.
- Use moisturizing wash rather than soap.
- Avoid extremes in temperature.
- Take an oatmeal bath (use colloidal oatmeal), which may provide soothing relief for dry, itchy skin. Oatmeal may help correct this by moisturizing and softening the skin, and providing protection against outside skin irritants.
- If your condition is severe, an eczema specialist may provide specific guidance on other bathing methods, such as a very mild bleach bath along with moisturizer treatments that may decrease bacteria on the skin, and reduce itchiness and discomfort associated with the condition. Consult with the specialist on the frequency and duration of these baths.
- Try phototherapy or ultraviolet (UV) light treatment, used in more severe cases. This involves exposure to artificial UVB and/

or UVA light several times a week, administered under a doctor's supervision.

. . . And by using some of these medications and other substances:

- Allergen-free massage oil (containing no fragrance or nut oil).
- Emollients and topical medications (or salves) that enhance skin moisture levels and attempt to correct the skin barrier defect responsible for moisture loss, a critical component in eczema. Emollients formulated as ointments (rather than creams) may be more effective for those with very dry skin; creams may be tolerated more broadly, and are often prescribed for use, twice daily.
- Topical steroids (both OTC and prescription) are very effective, and frequently the go-to topical treatment for mild to moderate eczema. In mild cases, low-dose potency topical steroids may start to work within days. In moderate to severe cases, a more potent topical steroid cream or ointment may be needed, and may require weeks before the full benefit is obvious. Prescription cor-

Thin-Skinned

Which area of the body is associated with the thinnest skin?

(a) arms   (b) back
(c) eyelids   (d) feet

The answer, of course, is (c), eyelids—along with the face, genitals, and skin folds. These areas may more readily absorb topical creams and medications; with that comes an increase in the risk of side effects. Overuse of strong cortisone on the eyelids could cause problems such as thinning of the skin, as well as cataracts and glaucoma.

When the Solution to the Problem
Is Another Problem

Danielle presented with breakouts on her face, and none of her OTC and prescription acne medications provided significant relief. She'd seen three dermatologists to no avail. The way her face looked made her feel ashamed; her self-esteem took a real hit. She told me she'd become a shut-in. I asked her some questions and then suggested a test to determine if she had any sensitivity to her skin care regimen. Patch testing pinpointed a skin allergy—to her acne medication regimen! We removed that treatment, found a new remedy to which she was not sensitive, and it finally started to work on the original problem. I created a "safe list" for her, which included the name of any major skin or acne care treatment that (a) was suitable for her condition and (b) did not contain the causative skin allergens. Within two to four weeks, Danielle had a fresh, beautiful, acne-free, blemish-free face.

The issue of acne can be confounding. There's a dizzying range of acne products out there, both OTC and prescription. As with Danielle's case, at times I see patients develop a rash, often to an ingredient in acne medication, which now worsens their facial concerns, since they've compounded acne with contact dermatitis or skin allergy to the products they went to for relief.

Alternatively, women who use lots of facial cosmetics, including cover-up or concealer, can have breakouts that they think is acne but isn't.

As an allergist, I am not the go-to specialist for acne—a dermatologist is better suited for that—but it's not uncommon for a patient's skin care regimen to be the cause of a rash or worse; and if she has sensitive skin, she may well react to an allergen in her acne preparation.

tisone creams are much stronger than OTC 1% hydrocortisone. However, potential side effects from long-term use, such as thinning of the skin, must be monitored by the patient and physician.

- Topical immunomodulators or calcineurin inhibitors to prevent flares; they are often used at the first sign of eczema, or for chronic eczema. They don't produce the side effects of cortisone.
- Antiseptic solutions, especially helpful in the event of skin infection.
- Tar solutions, to help reduce discomfort associated with inflammation.
- There are some new, exciting, not-yet-approved possibilities out there, including a biologic/injection and a nonsteroidal topical ointment, each of which has been touted for its apparent ability to block/reduce the inflammation of eczema.

Contact Dermatitis

This is a skin reaction—rash, blisters, itching, and burning—that follows contact with a substance. Contact dermatitis comes in two main types: irritant and allergic. Irritant contact dermatitis affects the outer skin almost exclusively. Redness, stinging, and/or itching can be caused by excessive dry or humid air; friction; soaps, alcohol, and other cleaning agents; and more. The irritant may cause the reaction by itself or in conjunction with other triggers. The offending substance is *not* an allergen (yet the immune system is actually also involved in irritant contact dermatitis). Examples of irritant contact dermatitis include chapped lips; "winter dry skin"; hand eczema from frequent hand-washing or chafing; and diaper rash (not all cases).

Allergic contact dermatitis involves a substance near or in contact with the skin that then triggers an immune reaction, which in turn causes red, itchy skin, among other symptoms. Examples of allergic contact dermatitis include poison ivy or poison oak dermatitis; a nickel reaction that causes a rash at the site of metal jewelry touching skin; a reaction to a personal care product (one or more components in the product), soap, detergent, shampoo, or fragrance; a chemical used in the workplace; certain plants; latex gloves; or medications.

Before the trigger is identified, near-term relief may often be found in a steroid cream. Your pharmacist can recommend a mild OTC topical corticosteroid, or your physician can prescribe one. Steroids control inflammation, and by reducing itchiness, reduce the need to scratch, enabling your skin to heal. (Helpful as such ointments are, a small percentage of patients may be allergic to the steroid cream. Skin patch testing can help determine if the solution is part of the problem.)

Individuals can be allergic to their clothes, specifically the formaldehyde resins that make fabrics waterproof, wrinkle-resistant, and shrink-resistant. Material like pure cotton, polyester, nylon, and acrylic are treated only lightly with resins. You also may be able to wear your favorite fabrics after they've been through the wash a lot. Wash them at least once before wearing for the first time, to reduce the chance of sensitization and developing a rash to the potential allergens found in permanent-press and wrinkle-resistant clothing and fabrics.

Is That Really a Wool Allergy or Are You Just Sensitive to Fiberglass?

The rash and itchiness caused by exposure to wool is actually the result of having sensitive skin. When seen under a microscope, wool looks like fiberglass. (Can you imagine how irritating a fiberglass shirt would feel, especially if you have sensitive skin?) The symptoms are likely the result of irritant contact dermatitis, not an allergic reaction. In fact, your response may not even be to the rough fibers of wool (though it might be) but to lanolin, an oil naturally found in wool, or to dyes and cleaning chemicals.

Cosmetics and Personal Care Products

On average, according to one study, a woman uses twelve types of personal-care products daily. Given the large number of substances and chemicals in each cosmetic, personal care product, and fragrance, both natural and artificial, it's no surprise that a considerable portion of the population experiences a reaction—sometimes allergic, sometimes not—during her lifetime. And that percentage may be low, since many of the reactions are mild, and often treated outside a doctor's intervention.

Some typical offenders:

- Facial cosmetics, lipstick, and eye shadow, which may contain nut oils and fragrances; and preservatives like parabens, quaternium-15 and, for aqueous-based cosmetics, a preservative that fights bacteria and fungal growth.
- Personal skin care products, which are overloaded with chemicals such as formaldehyde releasers; methyldibromo glutaronitrile, an allergen associated with hand dermatitis; and cocamidopropyl betaine, a surfactant that may cause a breakout on the eyelids, face, scalp or neck, and which is used often in shampoos, bath products, liquid shower gels, roll-on deodorants, liquid detergents, surface cleaners, pet care products, and other hair and skin care products.
- Nail polish—base coat, polish, top coat, or hardener—containing chemicals like formaldehyde resin and nickel mixing beads, which can lead to skin allergy from direct touching, particularly around the eyelids and eyes, which may cause puffiness/swelling, bumpy skin and other issues. While allergy to artificial nails is not common, some component in the nails or adhesives that make them stick may cause a reaction; if you're unsure about a potential problem, wear just one nail for a while to see if anything happens.
- Medications, which can include benzocaine, a sensitizer present in many OTC medications; and neomycin, a common antibacterial agent that can lead to allergic contact dermatitis.

Wait—It Wasn't My Eyeliner or Mascara?

■

A top cause of eyelid dermatitis? Nail polish. How so? The wearer touches her eye when the polish is still wet, enabling the active allergen to cause problems. Wait for it to dry.

FRAGRANCE

Fragrance was crowned Contact Allergen of the Year, an award bestowed by the American Contact Dermatitis Society, in 2007. It's a dubious honor, but one earned because fragrance is used in such a broad array of products, not just in fragrance, perfume, and cologne, but in other scented products such as cosmetics, medication, food, cleaning products, toothpaste, mouthwash, chewing gum, and mentholated cigarettes. It's estimated that 1 to 2 percent of the population has an allergy to fragrance, which is a leading cause of dermatitis. (Fragrance is responsible for 30 to 45 percent of atopic contact dermatitis in cosmetics.)

Fragrance allergy tends to present as a rash on the face, hands, and arms, or it may be generalized. Within hours of exposure, the affected area may turn red and swell intensely; in other instances, the rash may not appear until one or two weeks after exposure. Itchiness and dryness are other symptoms. Recommended treatment is topical corticosteroids and/or emollients, the same as for other types of acute dermatitis/eczema.

When we screen patients for "common sensitizers" in fragrance, we often patch test for something called "fragrance mix," a soup of eight distinct fragrances, each of which is a leading cause of fragrance allergy and each of which is used in numerous common products: alpha amyl cinnamic alcohol, cinnamaldehyde, cinnamyl alcohol, hydroxycitronellal, geraniol, isoeugenol, eugenol, and oak moss. A positive patch test to fragrance mix indicates that you're allergic to one or more fragrance

> ## Not What It Sounds Like It Means
>
> ■
>
> On a product label, "unscented" and "fragrance free" do *not* mean the product has zero fragrances. *Unscented* indicates no odor—likely because a fragrance is used to mask the not-so-great smell of other ingredients. If you're sensitive to the masking fragrance or one or more of the other chemicals in this "fragrance-free" product, you're likely to have a reaction.

chemicals. A patch test can identify the culprit for about three-quarters of all fragrance allergies.

Fragrance allergy tends to be lifelong, and to worsen with more exposure.

HAIR DYE, HENNA, AND PPD

A patient had developed an unusual, extremely itchy rash on her scalp soon after returning from attending a wedding. While there, someone was offering guests the chance to get temporary henna tattoos; my patient did, and we soon figured out that she had a sensitivity to paraphenylenediamine (PPD), a common component in hair dye and temporary tattoo ink. We resolved it easily—but unknowingly she had risked something far more serious (fortunately, without suffering consequences).

PPD, the active chemical ingredient in many permanent and semi-permanent hair dyes, gives a natural look, allows hair to be shampooed without de-coloring, and renders perming relatively easy. Although PPD is a potential allergen and/or irritant, the FDA allows hair dyes to contain PPD—up to a threshold. These dyes are considered safe so long as you follow the instructions.

The FDA does *not* allow PPD directly on the skin—but tattoo artists may use black henna that contains PPD (good for rapid drying and maintaining color). This henna is often unregulated; the paste may contain toxic levels of PPD. That means that if you have already developed a sensitivity to PPD (through use of a regulated hair dye, say), exposure to a product that's *un*regulated for PPD could possibly trigger a serious allergic reaction. Short of that, reactions to PPD include mild, stinging/burning irritation at the scalp, neck, forehead, ears, and/or upper eyelids; and skin that becomes red, swollen, itchy, blistered, dry, thickened, and/or cracked. Symptoms may appear immediately or within forty-eight hours. PPD can also cross-react with other compounds.

Allergic contact dermatitis triggered by PPD is not uncommon among hairdressers and cosmetologists. Because PPD is also a component in photocopying and printing inks, and various other occupational substances, those prone to PPD irritation or allergy include film developers, fabric/apparel buyers, textile industry workers, and tattoo artists. PPD problems may also arise for those who dye their hair often, and those close to them.

There are safer dyes that do not provide permanent coloring, such as vegetable rinse hair dyes. Before trying some of these, consider patch testing in a dermatologist's or allergist's office. To DIY, dab a small amount of dye behind your ear or on your inner elbow, leaving it to dry.

Our First Guess Is Often Wrong

■

A mustachioed patient came to my office with a rash around his mouth. He regularly dyed his mustache, and I suspected it was a PPD reaction. When I confirmed that his dye contained PPD, the diagnosis looked even more cut-and-dried.

It turns out he didn't have a PPD sensitivity: Ceasing the use of the dye did not help. In the end, I discovered the true cause of his problem: a preservative in his lip balm.

Follow the instructions that come with the dye; if you suspect the possibility of allergy or irritation to the product, consult first with a dermatologist and/or allergist.

Nickel and Other Metals

Twenty years ago, nickel allergy was hardly a "thing," at least in my practice. Now, in many countries, it's the number one cause of atopic contact dermatitis in children and adults; of those who are patch-tested, it has a very high prevalence rate. With the proliferation and constant use of mobile phones, and a rise in tattooing and body piercing, nickel has shot up the list of metals causing allergy, accounting for 95 percent of the metal allergy I now see.

Nickel (another Contact Allergen of the Year champ) is used in metal alloys; aside from some cell phones, other electronic devices and jewelry, it may commonly be a component in alkaline batteries, appliances, belt buckles, coins, construction tools, doorknobs, eyelash curlers, household utensils, keys, metal eyeglass frames, multivitamins, paper clips, razors, safety pins, scissors, thimbles, and zippers. When it's part of a nickel-steel alloy—as in stainless steel—nickel is sufficiently "bound" that it typically won't cause contact dermatitis; one possible exception is stainless steel cookware, where nickel may be released at cooking temperatures.

Janice was one of many patients whose facial rash turned out to be the result of nickel metal allergy. I tested the covering of her phone for the metal; it was positive. I had her apply a thin coating of clear nail polish over the metal area that would regularly touch her face—and her rash was soon gone. If the location of your rash coincides with mobile phone use, you might forgo a patch test and instead purchase a nickel test kit online for less than thirty dollars. The kit can quickly identify the presence of nickel in your phone, costume jewelry, or other metal-based accessories. If you can't avoid contact with nickel, either cover the nickel or use clear nail polish to coat (or bond) the metal, thus creating a physical barrier between the nickel and you.

Showing Their Mettle

■

More than two decades ago in Europe, limitations were placed on nickel in consumer products. Studies have shown a dramatic decrease there in nickel sensitization.

There are phones with nickel-free surfaces, too.

From 1996 to 1998, gold was named by the North American Contact Dermatitis Group as the number six allergen; three years later, gold was recognized as a major enough scourge and cause of allergic contact dermatitis that it was named 2001 Contact Allergen of the Year. Gold is now a known allergen, one that causes facial and eyelid dermatitis. While most of gold's allergic reactions are related to jewelry, gold dental appliances (crowns, bridges, dentures) can cause oral lesion.

And then there's this. Not long ago, a European woman in her mid-forties with apparent dermatitis came to my office. A patch test revealed a very strong reaction to gold, though she said she never wore gold jewelry. I was stumped . . . until I found out she loved to eat cakes and confections that were gold-laced.

Potassium chromate is used in tanning leather and making cement; exposure to chromate can cause atopic contact dermatitis. Aside from those in the leather and construction industries, who else might be susceptible to this allergy? Those wearing leather shoes in warmer weather/climates, since perspiration aids in the release of chromate.

The Patch Test

Requiring no injection, this test assesses whether your rash is allergic contact dermatitis. It is administered under the care of an allergist or dermatologist.

Before I schedule a patient for a patch test, I'll ask her to list what she did before the rash appeared, and to bring in products she regularly uses or comes in contact with—e.g., cosmetics, personal care products, perhaps substances used in her workplace. It's important to get as accurate and complete a list as possible; my experience is that less than half of patch-test patients recall all the things that might make them itch.

If after the test there's evidence of an allergic or irritant reaction at any site, we know what needs to be avoided. If there's no reaction, we've done the important job of ruling out certain possibilities.

Hives

Hives (medical term: *urticaria*) are red, itchy, swollen/raised bumps or welts on the skin, ranging in size and location on the body. They may be associated with an allergic reaction, but often their cause is not easily identifiable, especially when hives persist.

If the condition lasts for less than six weeks, it's acute urticaria; longer than that, it's chronic urticaria.

A related skin condition, angioedema, is a swelling of deeper skin layers (i.e., under the skin). Affected areas are often lips, tongue, eyelids, hands, and feet. Hives appear to afflict women more frequently than men; women in their thirties may be the likeliest to suffer.

Most cases are over within days to weeks. It's not unusual for hives to occur without easy explanation, then rarely, or maybe never, to recur. Less than 10 percent of hives cases are chronic.

ACUTE HIVES

It's said that if an allergic reaction results in hives or swelling, it was likely something that you ingested (food or an oral drug) or that was injected (drugs, venom from an insect sting), though acute hives may also be triggered by infection (viral or bacterial). When an allergen enters the bloodstream, a chain of events is set off in your immune system, culminating in the release of histamine, along with other chemicals. And voilà! You have hives (and possibly other symptoms).

Almost any allergen, in certain circumstances, can cause hives but some are particularly menacing:

Food allergens that commonly cause acute hives: The Big 8—egg, milk, peanut, tree nuts, fish, shellfish, wheat, soy. It's likelier that fresh food, not cooked, will cause hives when a food reaction occurs. While certain preservatives and food additives may be the cause, that's extremely rare.

Drugs: Antibiotics, such as penicillin; codeine and opiate-derived medications; aspirin and other NSAIDs. ACE inhibitors, for high blood pressure and cardiac care, can cause episodes of angioedema. The response to NSAIDs and ACE inhibitors is potentially life-threatening: The angioedema can result in dangerous swelling of the tongue and/or throat. Infrequently, topical products cause rash. An example of this is fragrance mix.

Venom: From insect stings—bee, yellow jacket, wasp, hornet, fire ant.

Oral antihistamines are recommended for treating acute episodes of hives. Injectable antihistamines and/or prescription steroid medication are sometimes needed for relief, especially in an urgent care setting, as well as epinephrine for anaphylaxis.

Hives can be caused by other factors—mostly physical but not always:

Cold. Itching, redness, and swelling occur quickly upon the skin's exposure to cold. It may be weeks after a viral infection before cold-induced urticaria expresses symptoms for the first time; they impact only the cold-exposed parts of the body.

Heat and/or exercise. Exertion, perspiring, high heat and humidity, and hot showers may each spark an outbreak; the trigger is typically a sudden change in body temperature. This may be known as cholinergic urticaria. The hives produced are small wheals (reddish, raised, and/or swollen marks on the skin). When the rash appears, it's a flushing of the neck and upper chest. It's extremely itchy. Gradually, the rash spreads to the back, face, and extremities. The wheals get bigger, too.

Exercise-induced hives is an uncommon condition but not rare, and there's a wide range of reactions. Exercise-induced anaphylaxis often presents with hives, swelling, and generalized itchiness, and may be accompanied (though, in my experience as a doctor, less frequently) by respiratory symptoms—trouble breathing, throat tightness, dizziness, and low blood pressure. The hives may be large; they may vary in size. A form of this condition—triggered by eating a particular food and exercising within a few hours—may lead to anaphylaxis.

Emotion, anxiety. Another form of cholinergic urticaria expresses itself as hives; the outbreak is the result of emotional responses.

Vibration or pressure. A rare form of hives and swelling known as vibratory urticaria, which occurs when extended pressure or vibration has been applied, resulting in swollen hands (from an activity like hammering or holding on to lawn mower handles); swollen feet (after walking); swollen buttocks (sitting for hours).

Sun. A rare disorder, sunlight-associated hives and itching emerge rapidly—within one to three minutes—after brief exposure to light. Swelling and redness of the exposed area follow. Within one to three hours, symptoms tend to disappear. A symptom of autoimmune disease is extreme sensitivity to the sun.

Water (aquagenic urticaria). After contact with water (regardless of temperature), small wheals develop on the skin. This condition is not common.

Medical conditions. The appearance of hives can signal one of several medical conditions, including thyroid disease or hepatitis.

For short-term relief, take antihistamine and/or anti-itch medication. If you're concerned that exposure to some substance or condition may cause hives, an allergist or dermatologist may prescribe an antihistamine prophylactically, to prevent or minimize the reaction (should it occur).

It's Always Sunny

■

Phytophotodermatitis—photoallergic contact dermatitis, or "sun sensitivity"—is a condition in which ultraviolet light (usually from the sun), in combination with a substance on the body, causes a reaction. One patient, a bartender, told me that he had repeatedly developed a red, itchy, unsightly rash on his fingers and hands after working parties. During an initial evaluation, a cause was not apparent. It looked somewhat like poison ivy (or poison oak or poison sumac). In taking his history, I discovered that a lot of his work took place outdoors during the summer, where he mixed lots of fruit- and citrus-based cocktails, particularly margaritas with lots of lime. We also uncovered that he frequently cut the fruits and prepared the drinks in sunny areas in the client's backyard, or in other exposed settings. His direct exposure to citrus, coupled with exposure to lots of sunlight, yielded the diagnosis of the relatively rare phytophotodermatitis. From then on, he did the same cutting and handling of the limes but indoors or without direct sun exposure. The problem disappeared.

Sometimes an allergen won't cause a skin reaction unless the skin is also exposed to sunlight. This condition can occur with products such as shaving lotion, sunscreen, and some perfumes.

CHRONIC HIVES

When hives and swelling last beyond six weeks, it's chronic hives/angioedema. In many cases, the exact cause eludes us. In some cases, your provider or specialist may order diagnostic blood testing to help determine a possible cause. In most cases, oral antihistamines and certain lifestyle changes can help to reduce and control symptoms. You may suffer from chronic hives for months or even years, with symptoms that wax and wane. We really want and need to understand more about this condition.

Dermographism

■

If stroking the surface of your skin causes a red line to develop, perhaps accompanied by swelling and/or itchiness, that's dermographism, which means "writing on the skin." Its cause is sometimes a mystery; it could be that histamine is released in response to the pressure on the skin, but it could also have another cause. Approximately 2 to 5 percent of the population, often young people, experience it. It may be triggered by exercise, friction, and after bathing. The simplest treatment is generally an oral antihistamine. In some cases, phototherapy provides benefit.

WHAT CAN HELP WITH HIVES (ASTHMA, TOO)?

Although hives—chronic hives, in particular—are a source of frustration for allergists and immunologists, they also represent an opportunity. We know that *something* is causing these breakouts of red, itchy welts on the skin. An autoimmune condition like lupus or thyroid disease? Latex rubber? An infection such as hepatitis? An insect bite or sting? A food or medication? Something else?

Aside from providing short-term relief—antihistamine and anti-itch medication and if those don't work, corticosteroids—what else can I do for my patients?

Data from my colleagues in neuroimmunology (yes, it's a specialty) report that heightened stress may impact certain skin conditions like eczema, seborrheic eczema, chronic urticaria, and pruritus. Theoretically, any engagement that reduces stress may be helpful—e.g., working with a therapist, doing yoga or exercise, or biofeedback. As yet, few studies support specific interventions aimed at reducing stress and anxiety. But the link between less stress and diminished hives is well documented.

I tend to assume that stress plays a role in some percentage of my patients' improved health profiles. As such, I encourage a "de-stress plan" made up of these elements:

1. *Yoga:* Although research says its benefits for asthma are limited, and its ability as primary prevention are unproven, yoga is practiced by some individuals looking for targeted improvement. One study found that the benefits of yoga on lung functioning were very small. There were some improvements with forms of yoga that emphasize breathing; for the most part, though, it was no more effective than standard breathing exercises. Colleagues of mine with large contingents of patients suffering from anxiety often recommend the Pranayama and Buteyko methods.

2. *Exercise:* Improves cardiac pulmonary fitness; swimming has shown improvement in asthma and lung function measurements.

3. *Meditation and relaxation* (including focused breathing, mindfulness meditation): Well-established antidotes to stress, they often work to reduce or eliminate hives, less so in improving asthma. Urticaria-chronic relaxation therapy addresses underlying emotional problems and outside factors that can worsen eczema and cause hives. (As noted earlier, it's common for me to see hives outbreaks shortly after a major stressor in the patient's life.) New subfields addressing this connection are psychoneuroimmunology and psychodermatology.

4. *Biofeedback:* Versus placebo, heart-rate-variability biofeedback has been shown it may lead to better lung function, fewer symptoms, and reduction in medication.

5. *Improved sleep:* Studies show that improved sleep quality is associated with better asthma control; napping may be more associated with individuals, particularly children, with asthma. (Daytime napping in children is an indication that more quality nighttime sleep is needed; this deserves attention, especially in asthmatics.)

6. *Family therapy:* For children suffering from allergy and asthma, this may be a beneficial adjunct to medication.

Allergy Masquerade

■

It's said that to a man with a hammer, everything looks like a nail. It's important for us allergists to remember that not everything that looks like allergy is allergy.

Swollen elbow, swollen feet, swollen hands: While Miranda's condition resembled a possible allergic reaction to a food, drug, or another trigger, it turned out not to be that at all.

It was a surprising diagnosis.

After taking a careful history of Miranda's background, I uncovered that a month before, she had been on a weeklong hiking trip. I ordered a blood test—which confirmed that she had Lyme disease, the cause of the swelling.

A reminder: Not everything that swells is allergy.

Poison Ivy

As with other allergens, if you are wired to be allergic to poison ivy, you won't break out the first time. You need to be exposed to it at least once (and often many times) for the horrible itchiness, redness, irritation, etc., to kick in.

We know all the things we hate about poison ivy (and poison oak and poison sumac). Before it is washed off, the plant's oil, urushiol (or "rhus oil"), spreads to cause that horrible rash, which swells into blistering, incredibly itchy pimples, which often morph into larger, orange, dome-shaped blisters.

It takes only one-billionth of a gram of urushiol to set off an allergic reaction that is so often a misery. And even after the poison ivy plant has died, its oil can remain active for years. No plant accounts for more doctor and ER visits. But for all that unpleasant information, here's some even more daunting news: Thanks in part to climate change, poison ivy is now in even more places than it was. Over the last half century, the plant has exploded in volume and potency. Leaves the size of pie pans are not atypical. As carbon dioxide levels rise, and pass new, disturbing thresholds, poison ivy's growth is predicted to continue skyrocketing.

What to do with this distressing news?

Presumably, there's an ever-expanding commercial opportunity for some enterprising individual to come up with more treatment options or a prevention protocol. For now, Tecnu soap and Ivy Block may remove the nasty and stubborn urushiol before the eruption of rash. Some products can keep urushiol from reaching the skin. Certain dishwashing soaps (e.g., Dial Ultra) may help to remove the skin of urushiol before the allergic reaction takes place.

If You Can Conveniently Keep Allergens Out of the Home, Do

Ted stored his golf clubs in the house, near the couch in the den. His kids routinely used all the space in the room for their play activities—and then his younger son, Henry, got a small rash that, within a couple of days, exploded into a blistering rash on the legs. His folks took him to a dermatologist, who gave Henry a topical steroid cream—and all was solved.

Until the following month, when, several days after Ted's country club golf tournament, Henry again developed a rash, this one so bad that he wound up in urgent care for treatment. I saw them soon after that, when they were investigating the possibility of allergy. I'd asked them to bring some photographs of the house—outside and in—and after looking at the pictures and asking a few questions, it became obvious: Ted's golf clubs, in the den. When he returned from playing golf, they were covered with urushiol. I told Ted to keep the golf bag, clothing, and accessories in the garage and out of the house, away from areas where the kids frequented.

Mango, No Go

∎

Urushiol, the nasty oil in poison ivy and poison oak, is also found in the oil of mango sap. This is no surprise, since mangoes are part of the large cashew family, which also includes poison oak, poison ivy, and poison sumac. While those who react to urushiol can usually eat mango without problem (urushiol isn't found in the flesh of the fruit), touching the mango skin, or the leaves or bark of the mango tree, may lead to itching, hives, redness, and blisters within a day or two.

If you are fighting a bout of poison ivy, avoid eating cashews because it may prolong symptoms.

If you are suffering, try to calm the itch and rash with topical steroid cream or ointment, available usually with a prescription. I also recommend using an ice compress to relieve itching. If itching is severe, antihistamines and oral prednisone may be recommended.

Sunscreen Allergy and Sun Sensitivity

The effectiveness of sunscreens has improved dramatically in the last few decades. Years ago, before the rise in awareness of skin cancer and skin damage, and before the effects of our vanishing ozone layer, which protects us from the sun's ultraviolet rays, there was little urgency that such a form of sun protection was needed. When sunscreen came to popularity, the protection provided was equivalent to, approximately, SPF 4 to 8; today, use an SPF under 30, and your beachmates will think you're reckless. The American Academy of Dermatology (AAD) encourages sunscreen use for several reasons, including helping to lower the risk of skin cancer, sunburn, and signs of aging.

If your use of sunscreen, or another product in the sun, leads to rash, a patch test administered by a dermatologist or allergist might be very useful. It should pinpoint the culprit, be it sunscreen agent, fragrance, preservative, or something else.

SUNSCREEN: PHYSICAL OR CHEMICAL?

It's ironic perhaps that a topical product you use to protect your skin can itself cause an unwanted skin reaction. How do you know which of the many available sunscreens work best for you? (Use of the word "sunblock" has been banned for such products; they are all called "sunscreen" so there is no false sense of security that all UV rays are being blocked.) There are two categories: physical sunscreens and chemical (or organic) sunscreens (or absorbers). The former contain active mineral ingredients (e.g., titanium dioxide or zinc oxide) that deflect/scatter UV rays. The latter contain organic compounds (benzophenone, oxybenzone, octinoxate, octisalate, avobenzone) that create a chemical reaction and transform UV rays into heat, which is then released from the skin.

Below are the pros and cons of the two types of sunscreen:

PROS OF PHYSICAL SUNSCREEN

- Broad spectrum—both UVA and UVB protection
- No delay in effect—immediate protection after application
- Water resistant
- Less irritating for sensitive skin
- No sensitization reported
- Preferred for those with rosacea and tendency to flush, and often better tolerated in those of sensitive skin types
- Better for acne-prone skin
- Longer shelf life

CONS OF PHYSICAL SUNSCREEN

- Can leave white film on skin, making it more visible
- Need to spread evenly to be effective
- Can feel thick and heavy

PROS OF CHEMICAL SUNSCREEN

- Easier to apply, less thick than physical screens
- Easier to combine with skin-enhancing antioxidants and vitamin additives

CONS OF CHEMICAL SUNSCREEN

- Need to apply twenty minutes prior to sun exposure to be effective
- More chemicals needed for both UVA and UVB protection, which can lead to more skin irritation and/or sensitivity
- Can run into eyes, leading to irritation
- Can clog pores, leading to acne
- Must be reapplied often
- More common cause of allergic contact dermatitis

Latex

Years ago, a patient complained of a generalized rash, occasionally hives, she would experience during or after shifts working at the restaurant her family owned. By the time Bonnie came to see me, it had happened at least five times: Each time, she'd sought relief from a nearby urgent care facility, was prescribed antihistamines, oral steroids, and topical steroids cream, and the problem went away—until the next time. We went through a number of possibilities but an immediate answer did not present itself. Then a blood test came back showing that Bonnie had an off-the-chart level of allergic sensitivity to latex rubber. The kitchen staff, I discovered, wore latex rubber gloves while cutting and prepping vegetables for lunches and dinners. We switched the staff gloves to non-latex, and Bonnie experienced no more recurrences.

This is perhaps the lone type of allergic reaction that I've seen *less* of in the last decade. Many establishments, especially hospitals, doctors' offices, and other employers of health care workers have switched to gloves that are non-latex or low-protein latex.

An allergy to latex may develop after repeated exposure to medical gloves, balloons, or other latex-based products; if you often have an itchy mouth after dental exams, you may well have a latex allergy. Asthma symptoms may accompany more extreme cases. Note that direct physical contact need not occur; that was almost certainly the case with Bonnie, where airborne particles from the powder of the gloves might have been enough to trigger her reaction.

Because of the concept of cross-reactivity (see chapter 8), you can develop a latex allergy without ever having encountered latex. The proteins in latex are very similar to those in avocado, edible chestnuts, fig, kiwi, mango, papaya, passion fruit, pineapple, potatoes, and more; if you've developed an allergic sensitization to one of these related foods, your immune system may react to latex, "thinking" it's the offending protein.

It's important to note that allergy to latex is considerably less common than an irritant reaction—from wearing latex gloves, for example—or a "delayed-type" allergic reaction.

Myth: Avoid Latex Paint If You Have a Latex Allergy

■

Untrue: Latex paint does not contain natural latex rubber, the common allergen. Why the name of the paint? Latex house paint is made from chemicals, including synthetic rubber latex, which is not known to cause allergic reaction. Natural rubber latex does trigger allergic responses in many people—but it's not a component of latex paint.

Lovemaking and Intimacy

What we wear on our bodies and put into them can affect not merely ourselves but also others with whom we have close contact, especially skin to skin. Your partner may experience a skin reaction—redness, irritation, hives—to the facial product, fragrance, or cosmetic you're wearing. You may react to the shaving cream or other facial product your partner is wearing. Presuming kissing is involved, you should avoid— for sixteen to twenty-four hours before physical intimacy—any food or medication known to cause an allergic reaction or irritation in your partner. Toothbrushing and mouth rinsing to eliminate any trace of potential food allergen helps but only to a point: Allergens can remain in saliva for up to twenty-four hours, post-ingestion. Common allergic outbreaks to kissing include swelling of the lips or throat, hives, rash, itching, and wheezing.

Spermicides, lubricants, and/or latex condoms may contain chemicals that cause allergic reaction. Latex-free condoms are available. Seminal plasma allergy—an adverse reaction to the protein in semen within minutes of intercourse—is an extremely rare condition; in a study of women who were susceptible to it, more than three-quarters of them had a history of other allergies (pollen, food). While sperm allergy reportedly affects mostly women, another condition, post-orgasmic illness syndrome (POIS), occurs in men, who may experience common cold-like, generalized symptoms that may last for days. Although this condition is uncommon, one European study found that 88 percent of men tested positive for sensitivity to their semen.

Insect Bites and Stings

See chapter 5, Outdoor and Seasonal Allergies.

Chapter 8

Food Allergies

■

Awareness of food allergy is rising. But is the rate of food allergy rising, too? I suspect so. I say "suspect" because there has not been a robust updated collection of food allergy rates on a global scale, and most of the data we do have are from just the United States and Europe. I also believe, as referenced in chapter 1, that the globalization of food and our greater individual mobility, among other factors, may have led to more food allergy, diagnosed and not.

But some researchers aren't so sure. They estimate that only one-quarter of those who believe they have a food allergy actually do, that many of these individuals are more likely to have food intolerance, such as lactose intolerance, than a food allergy. (Initial diagnosis is complicated because food intolerance often presents with symptoms similar to a food allergy, including abdominal complaints.) We need to be aware that there's a difference between a reported food allergy—where the individual has a history of eating a particular food and experiencing typical allergic symptoms—and allergy that's diagnosed by testing. If you suspect a food allergy in yourself or your child, get evaluated by an experienced allergist.

Food allergy means exposure, through ingestion, to a food that triggers an immune system reaction whose symptoms range from mild to severe to potentially fatal. A ten-year longitudinal survey reported that the prevalence of (self-reported) food allergy had increased among US adults, from 2001 to 2010. According to a survey cited by the Centers for Disease Control and Prevention, the incidence of food allergy among children in the United States rose by half between 1997 and 2011. One often-cited study by Dr. Hugh Sampson, one of the country's foremost experts in pediatric food allergy, surveyed kids in the 1980s; when testing a comparable cohort a decade later, he discovered that the existence of antibodies to peanut—one of the Big Eight food allergens—had risen by 55 percent, while allergic reactions had nearly doubled. Another study (albeit one by no means perfect in its methodology) showed that, from 1997 to 2008 (as reported at three intervals in a phone survey of households), the rate of peanut allergy more than tripled in US children. While allergies to milk, egg, wheat, and soy tend to resolve during childhood, they may be resolving slower than previously: One extensive source revealed that, in certain cases, kids remain allergic past age five and into their teenage years. Incidence of severe reaction may be on the rise, too, as food allergy is the number one cause of anaphylaxis outside hospitals. Over six million US adults are allergic to shellfish or finned fish.

Nor is this just an American phenomenon. Food allergy may be rising in other countries, too. In Europe, the last decade has seen a 700 percent rise in hospital admissions of children with severe food allergy reactions.

Treatment for Severe Reaction to Food Allergy

A serious reaction can be controlled by epinephrine, part of an emergency plan. Antihistamines may often control milder symptoms, but epinephrine should always be available because even mild symptoms can progress into more severe ones.

With food allergy comes other vulnerabilities and complications. Food-allergic kids are two to four times likelier to suffer from asthma and/or other allergies, including hay fever, than those without; respiratory allergies in general are about three times more prevalent among food-allergic kids. It's believed that having a family history of food allergy increases your likelihood of developing eczema, and vice versa.

Why the apparent rise in certain food allergies? To be honest, we're not absolutely sure. Environment may play a role: Some think it has contributed meaningfully to altering the makeup of our intestinal microbiota—today more popularly known as gut bacteria—which is crucial to immune system development and overall health. It may be that the lower rates of infection during childhood, or the increased reliance on antibiotics and hand sanitizers, may shift the type of bacteria that occurs naturally in the gut; researchers have shown that these bacteria may shield us from food allergen sensitization, a precursor to developing actual food allergy.

Other explanations for a rise in food allergy include greater awareness (the Girl Scouts of America now have a special merit badge for members who develop an understanding of food allergy that can be valuable to food-allergic friends) to introduction of certain foods at younger ages, before the full development of the immune system, to *avoidance* of foods at younger ages, when resistance may develop.

There's also the tricky nature of the condition. A food allergy is a "hypersensitivity" reaction, the result of exposure to an allergen in a particular food. This is a tightly defined immunologic reaction involving the susceptible individual, a specific protein, a specific antibody, and symptoms provoked from ingestion. Or you may react only to a food in its raw or uncooked state, particularly a fruit or vegetable, a condition known as oral allergy syndrome or pollen-food syndrome (more on this on page 208). In exceedingly rare circumstances, you may react to a food allergen when exposed to it via skin contact or inhalation—e.g., breathing in the steam of shellfish that's being boiled. (This route of reaction has been alleged but never proven in a handful of studies on peanuts.)

A Matter of When

■

I noted that a possible explanation for the rise in food allergy is the introduction of food to those whose immune system is not yet mature enough to "handle" it; or, conversely, that certain foods were eliminated (if for well-meaning reasons) from the very early diet. In both cases, the "when" could matter. If the hygiene hypothesis is correct, then we weaken the development of the immune system by shielding it from "invaders" early on. A recent study explored the development of diabetes and the accompanying destructive response of the immune system in Russian, Finnish, and Estonian newborns. The researchers concluded that improved hygiene kept the infants from being exposed to common infections, which in turn may be responsible for the rate of autoimmune diseases. Perhaps the same is true with certain potential food allergens.

Too Much on the Menu

Food-allergic reactions are very often simply unpredictable. As researchers Amy M. Branum and Susan L. Lukacs wrote bluntly in their 2008 study on food allergy among children in the United States: "The mechanisms by which a person develops an allergy to specific foods are largely unknown." Food allergies appear to behave more aggressively and unpredictably than they once did. "We may be dealing with a different kind of disease process than we did twenty years ago," says one doctor. We can't say for sure why this is happening. But we also lack great data from the past, because food allergy was poorly recognized.

Many foods and food components are known potential allergens, yet there are more out there to be discovered, as well as more food allergen combinations, and food allergen/non-food allergen combos. There is a dizzying array of classifications for adverse food reactions. Do you or your child have gluten intolerance or celiac disease, or lactose intolerance or milk allergy? Is it peach that you can't eat—or peach in combination with your preexisting hay fever? Is that peanut oil or soybean oil safe only when it's refined and/or hydrogenated and/or partially hydrogenated?

It's complicated.

We know this: Food allergy has yet to be cured. We know that some food allergies resolve, and do so early on. We know that major food allergens, such as cow's milk, egg, wheat, and soy, are more common in children under age five. We believe that certain kinds of allergy, particularly oral allergy syndrome, are more common in adults than children. We know that once the food culprit is recognized, strict avoidance is recommended—but that's often not easy, even for the most vigilant individual or parent of a food-allergic child. It can be exhausting and frightening to have food allergy, or to be the parent or caregiver of a food-allergic child, especially when considering that almost half of fatal food allergy reactions (though uncommon) are triggered by food consumed outside the home. Even if you do avoid the offending food(s), you may want to replace it with other sources of important nutrients so that malnourishment is not a potential issue.

In this chapter, I examine the various food allergies and how they are best diagnosed, averted, and managed. A useful food allergy action plan is based on the following:

- Confirm the diagnosis.
- Get informed, which includes learning the signs and symptoms of a food reaction.
- Understand ingredient labels.
- Avoid food allergen exposure.
- Prepare a medical alert.
- Carry a chef ingredient card.
- Have on-hand availability and knowledge of the proper use of an epinephrine auto-injector.

First, though, some much-needed definitions.

Don't Overtest

■

If a child has a food allergy, will his or her sibling have one? For some time, it was simply thought that, yes, the chance was quite high, which meant siblings were often being needlessly tested—and misdiagnosed. However, a 2016 study showed that just one in eight kids with a food-allergic sibling also had a food allergy (slightly more than half the siblings had positive food tests but could still eat the food in question). The finding is important in helping to reduce needless screening. Food testing is currently recommended for siblings only to help confirm a suspected diagnosis of food allergy after a reaction, not to establish its existence. (As allergists, we do not have a crystal ball.) One study showed that 9 percent of kids tested positive for peanut allergies, yet just 1 percent developed allergic reaction attributed to eating peanuts. If your child develops hives after consuming a peanut butter cookie and has no history with peanut products, it makes sense to have her tested for peanut allergy; it does not make sense to test her for wheat allergy, if she has previously eaten wheat without problems, or has never eaten wheat and you're curious to know if she might be allergic. Allergy tests are not designed to predict the future. They are best used to confirm a history of reported reaction.

Defining Our Terms

Not every adverse reaction to food is a food allergy. Most are not, and as noted earlier, an allergy implies a very specific immunologic reaction. Yet many people, including physicians, use *allergy* as an umbrella term. Still, vocabulary matters. Some responses occur in everyone, under certain eating conditions, like eating spoiled food: This is not an allergy. Some responses occur, generating symptoms that look like allergy, but in fact the immune system is not in overdrive; this, too, is not an allergy but evidence (to take one example) of the lack of a crucial enzyme—e.g., what happens when a lactase-deficient individual consumes milk. It's key for us as doctors, and you as a consumer of health knowledge, to know the differences. The diagnostic strategies we choose depend on what we believe the problem to be.

FOOD SENSITIZATION

This really means "risk for a certain food." Simply, your body produces the antibody IgE against that particular food. For example, you may have eaten tomatoes all your life without issue. However, if you took a skin test for tomato, you might see a small red bump on your arm showing that you have likely developed sensitization to tomato. Your body has produced tomato-specific IgE antibodies. Yet, importantly, *this does not mean that you are allergic to tomato and must stop eating it.* After all, you've eaten it without incident, and thus don't have an allergy to it, by definition. This is the hard part about testing "positive": With many other disease states, a positive test means disease. Not so with allergy. Sensitization is very common, and often misinterpreted as allergy—but (again) allergy is more than sensitization. It is sensitization in someone who develops real-world symptoms to that food.

Why would someone have a positive test and yet be tolerant? That is

When Reading Labels Is Not Enough

In one study of food allergy, the majority of reactions were triggered by accidental exposure to foods the person had considered safe: Either she unintentionally ate a food to which she was allergic; misread a label; or the food she ate was cross-contaminated—while being prepared, stored, or served—with a food to which she was allergic.

The Age of Vulnerability

■

Those at greatest risk of food-induced anaphylaxis fatalities? Food-allergic teens and food-allergic young adults. Why might this be? My guess is that they're part of the cohort likeliest not to carry around their epinephrine auto-injectors: They take big risks; they think they're invincible; or maybe they're concerned about being made fun of or ostracized.

unclear. In practical terms, there's little difference between someone who has a sensitivity to a food and is tolerant of it, and someone who has no sensitivity at all.

FOOD ALLERGY

A food allergy is an abnormal, time-limited immune system response to a food protein that expresses itself with very characteristic symptoms. Usually (but not always), the allergen is a naturally occurring protein, and the body treats it (if falsely, thanks to evolution) as a serious threat. An allergic reaction to even a very small amount of a food can occur; the great majority of the population can consume this food, in ample quantity, without problem. For those who are allergic, the reaction will be immediate, with symptoms presenting within minutes of ingestion— such as a child's mouth swelling and throat itching very soon after eating peanuts.

Certain allergens trigger a reaction mostly when the particular food—primarily fruits and vegetables—is consumed in its raw form. This is oral allergy syndrome or pollen-food syndrome (see page 208).

Symptoms of an acute food-allergic reaction may include one or more of the following: tingling/swelling of the lips, tongue, mouth, throat; itching of tongue/throat; throat tightness; hives, general itchiness; stomach cramps/abdominal pain, vomiting, diarrhea; wheezing, shortness of breath; dizziness/feeling faint, loss of consciousness; and, in rare circumstances, death.

In young children, food allergy may worsen eczema, particularly a severe case.

FOOD INTOLERANCE

"Intolerance" is a catch-all term: It means simply that you don't "tolerate" a particular food. Unlike an allergy, this is not an immune-mediated reaction, even though symptoms may overlap. Enzyme deficiency is a common cause of food intolerance. For example, if you're lactose-intolerant, you don't possess the enzyme lactase, which is required to digest milk sugar. When you consume milk or milk products, you may experience symptoms like gas, bloating, abdominal pain, and diarrhea.

There is a test for confirming intolerance to lactose or fructose.

TOXIC REACTIONS TO FOOD

These reactions, such as food poisoning, can be caused by bacteria, viruses, or parasites. They differ from food allergy in that virtually anyone who ingests such contaminated food will suffer symptoms.

These reactions occur from either direct human transmission of bacteria or viruses to the food (from improper hygiene) or improper handling and storage of food. Staphylococcal food poisoning is fairly common and manifests as acute gastroenteritis. (Yes, you can go ahead and blame it on your aunt's potato salad that sat out at the picnic too long.) It can also happen after consuming fish of a certain species, such as tuna, mackerel, or mahimahi, that have been stored at insufficiently cool temperatures and spoiled: Histamine is produced in the fish, you ingest it, and your symptoms mimic an allergic reaction; this is called scombroid poisoning. While "intoxications" are not food allergies, they may be confused with them because of a similar range of symptoms—redness, itchiness, hives, GI upset, nausea, and vomiting.

The good news? While we hear now and then about an outbreak of

Food Condition	Definition	Symptoms	Diagnosis	Treatment
Food Allergy	An immediate immune system response to a protein in a particular food. Can be life-threatening.	Hives, swelling, cramping, vomiting, shortness of breath, wheezing, coughing, trouble swallowing, dizziness, anaphylaxis.	An allergist or immunologist can perform a skin prick test and/or blood test and, if indicated, an oral food challenge.	Avoid offending food(s) completely.
Food Intolerance	An adverse response to food that does not involve the immune system. Can have a number of causes, including lack of an enzyme required for proper digestion of a food.	Vomiting, cramping, bloating, distention, gas, diarrhea, constipation, and reflux—to name a few.	A GI specialist can perform breath tests for lactose intolerance (and sometimes fructose malabsorption). For other suspected intolerances, a registered dietitian can guide an elimination diet to identify trigger foods.	Avoid large quantities of offending food(s) or food components. Small quantities may be tolerated. Note: For lactose intolerance, enzyme tablets or modified dairy foods can be taken.
Celiac Disease	An autoimmune condition in which the body attacks gluten, and is immunologic in nature—thus, it is NOT an intolerance.	Malabsorption, diarrhea, abdominal distention, bloating and discomfort, weight loss in children, and associated symptoms.	Screening blood tests, such as tTG-IgA test, are commonly used.	The only treatment at present is a gluten-free diet.
Toxic Reactions to Food	Otherwise known as food poisoning. Often bacterial, parasitic, and/or viral infection, due to poor hygiene, handling, and/or processing of suspect food(s). Histamine fish poisoning/toxin. Not an allergy.	Typical symptoms of acute, sudden onset of familiar gastrointestinal complaints, such as vomiting, fever, and diarrhea. Often leads to dehydration.	In mild cases, diagnostic tests are not commonly done. In more severe episodes, blood and stool tests can pinpoint specific toxins responsible for symptoms.	Be vigilant, especially during hot weather; food items exposed for prolonged periods and/or not properly handled.

E. coli or a similar contaminant, food preparation today is more hygienic than ever.

The Hateful 8

About 90 percent of food-allergic reactions are caused by eight types of food :

- Cow's milk
- Hen's egg
- Peanut
- Tree nuts (almond, walnut, cashew, hazelnut, Brazil nut, pistachio, pecan)
- Fin fish
- Shellfish (both soft-shell crustacean and hard-shell mollusk)
- Wheat
- Soy

The Food Allergen Labeling and Consumer Protection Act (FALCPA) of 2004 mandates specific labeling requirements for these eight foods.

How Tolerant Are You?

When speaking of an allergy, *tolerate* connotes one of two related conditions: You have naturally outgrown your allergy; or you have received therapy that has successfully prevented symptoms from developing, after you are exposed to the allergen in question. Tolerance may be short-term or long-term. For food allergy, there are no approved treatments at present, though these are under investigation. Tolerance is subjective but involves you being able to eat the particular food any time, in any quantity.

Alcohol: Probably Intolerance, Rarely Allergy

■

Is it the amaretto—or the almonds in it? If you don't feel great after drinking a bit, is potential allergy really the reason?

Alcohol intolerance—the phrase is often used interchangeably with "alcohol allergy" but as with food, the descriptors do mean different things—triggers an immediate, unpleasant reaction after you drink: Symptoms may include a runny/stuffy nose, facial redness, hives, nausea, vomiting, diarrhea, and worsening of preexisting asthma. The intolerance may be genetic: The body lacks the enzyme to break down alcohol's toxins into acetic acid or vinegar. This condition is often found in individuals of Asian descent (the prevalence may be as high as 70 percent among those of Han Chinese descent); it is sometimes referred to as "Asian flush." Unfortunately, the lone way to truly prevent alcohol intolerance–type reactions is simply to not drink alcohol.

European researchers have shown that some individuals (not many) have a likely allergic sensitivity to proteins present in grapes, thus wine.

Of the eight food categories, the ones attributed to causing the most fatal or near-fatal reactions are peanuts and tree nuts. However, if you're allergic, any food can be associated with a severe reaction. There are no "soft" food allergies and no hierarchy whereby one allergen is "worse" than another. It's all relative and very personal.

If you have a food allergy: Aside from avoiding the food in question, what other approaches help you to live more freely? Oral immunotherapy—in which small amounts of food allergen, then increasing amounts, are administered for the purpose of desensitizing your food allergy—may have potential. It is not yet an approved or established therapy for food; despite promising preliminary studies that it may produce some benefit in some patients, more research is needed to clarify the scale of the therapy's benefit, its ideal target, and its safety. And a promising potential treatment for peanut allergy may be on the horizon: Some researchers have reported that this "peanut patch" may receive approval as early as 2018.

THE CHANCES OF OUTGROWING FOOD ALLERGY

The incidence of children affected by food allergy is much higher during the first year of life. For children younger than 5 years old, the rate is reported to be 6 to 8 percent; it's estimated that the total prevalence of food allergy among children and adolescents (from birth to age 17) is approximately 5.1 percent. Among adults, the prevalence worldwide is thought to be 3 to 4 percent.

Some food-allergic children will outgrow their conditions. How long it takes varies by person as well as food: It is far less common for food-allergic children to develop a tolerance for peanuts, tree nuts, or shellfish than for milk, egg, soy, or wheat.

On average, the younger the age of first food allergen reaction, the greater the likelihood the child will outgrow the allergy. Over time, the antibody level may rise or fall (usually the latter); in general, the lower the level, the greater the chance the individual will pass an oral food challenge.

If a child has multiple food allergies, she is less likely to outgrow one or all of them. According to an extensive 2016 study, a food-allergic child has a 35 percent chance of developing asthma. On a happier note, children appear capable of still outgrowing food allergy later than previously thought—during adolescence and even beyond. (The findings of this study at Johns Hopkins Children's Hospital were taken from children with more persistent, severe food allergies than the general population.)

Both blood tests and skin tests, followed serially over time, can help an allergist assess the likelihood that a child will outgrow her food allergy. A changing number in yearly blood tests can provide guidance for forecasting the allergy's duration. Given that kids can outgrow food allergy well into the teen years and young adulthood, they should be encouraged to get properly evaluated by an allergist to see if they have finally outgrown it. I've had numerous adult patients who had been allergic to a food for years when growing up, and believed they still were—until a test suggested that the level of recognition had waned significantly (and they may have been depriving themselves of the food for many years).

MILK[1]

The number one food allergy in infants and young kids, milk allergy frequently develops in the first year of life, and most children outgrow it. An allergy to cow's milk generally indicates allergy to the milk of other domestic animals (e.g., goat, sheep, etc.), whose milk protein is similar and may cross-react in over 95 percent of cases.

The terms "nondairy" and "dairy-free" are not limited by FALCPA, and milk derivatives such as caseinates may be ingredients in foods labeled "nondairy." It is required, however, that caseinates be listed among the ingredients, followed by "(milk)."

Most children who are allergic to cow's milk are able to tolerate baked milk. An allergist can help provide specific guidance and instructions for your child.

AVOIDANCE LIST

- Butter, butter fat, butter oil, butter acid, butter ester(s)
- Buttermilk
- Casein
- Cheese
- Cottage cheese
- Cream
- Curds
- Custard
- Diacetyl

---

1. Details about the Big 8 food allergens: ©2016, Food Allergy Research & Education. Adapted and used with permission.

- Ghee
- Half-and-half
- Lactalbumin, lactalbumin phosphate
- Lactoferrin
- Lactose
- Lactulose
- Milk (in all forms, including condensed, derivative, dry, evaporated, goat's milk and milk from other animals, low-fat, malted, milk-fat, nonfat, powder, protein, skimmed, solids, whole)
- Milk protein hydrolysate
- Pudding
- Recaldent
- Rennet casein
- Sour cream, sour cream solids
- Sour milk solids
- Tagatose
- Whey (in all forms)
- Whey protein hydrolysate
- Yogurt

Does This Have Milk (Technically, Milk Protein)? Nope—You're Good.

■

- Calcium lactate
- Calcium stearoyl lactylate
- Cocoa butter
- Cream of tartar
- Lactic acid (lactic acid starter culture may contain milk)
- Oleoresin
- Sodium lactate
- Sodium stearoyl lactylate

Milk is *sometimes* found in:

* Artificial butter flavor
* Baked goods
* Caramel candies
* Chocolate
* Lactic acid starter culture and other bacterial cultures
* Luncheon meat, hot dogs, sausages
* Margarine
* Nisin
* Nondairy products
* Nougat

Though by no means likely, milk may be found in the following:

* Deli meat slicers, which are often used for both meat and cheese products.

Milk's Nutrients, Without the Milk

■

Since the nutrients we get from milk are valuable, what do you do for the food-allergic child? Try casein-hydrolysate formulas (Alimentum and Nutramigen are two such brands), which are extensively hydrolyzed, so that the protein has been "broken down" to differ from milk protein, thus less likely to trigger a reaction. These formulas are generally tolerated in milk-allergic children; however, in a small percentage of children they are not tolerated.

Soy-based formula is also recommended (so long as the infant is not also allergic to soy). These formulas are good sources of valuable nutrients, and are recommended beyond age one, for food-allergic kids on restricted diets.

Kosher Dairy

■

On the label of kosher products, the existence of milk protein—or at least the potential "contamination" by milk protein—is advertised by "D" or the word "dairy" following the circled K or U.

"Milk-free"—by the standards of kosher dietary law—is advertised by the word *pareve*. However, a product may be labeled "pareve" *yet still contain a minimal amount of milk protein*. For safety's sake, you may need to avoid these, too.

- Some brands of canned tuna fish contain casein, a milk protein/derivative; some meats may contain casein as a binder; many nondairy products contain casein. Check labels. Some specialty products made with milk substitutes (i.e., soy-, nut-, or rice-based dairy products) are manufactured on equipment shared with milk.

- Shellfish is sometimes dipped in milk to reduce the fishy odor.

- Many restaurants put butter on steaks after they have been grilled to add extra flavor. The butter is not visible after it melts.

- Some medications contain milk protein though it's unclear if this represents any harm. One expert recently reviewed this question, namely: What is the risk of a milk-allergic individual ingesting a milk protein or milk sugar in a pharmaceutical agent (OTC or prescription drug)? Reports of individuals experiencing an allergic reaction in such cases appear to be rare. On very rare occasions, contamination by cow's milk protein was found in some medications containing lactose.

EGG (HEN)

Egg allergy is the second-most common food allergy in kids. By age sixteen, in one study, more than two in three children had outgrown their egg allergy.

Although it's the white of the egg that contains the proteins (e.g., ovalbumin, ovotransferrin, lysosome, and ovomucoid) that are potentially allergenic, individuals with egg allergy should also avoid the yolk, given the difficulty in cleanly and fully separating white from yolk (cross-contact).

Like milk, egg is an allergen susceptible to high heat, and 70 to 80 percent of egg-allergic individuals tolerate "baked egg." Tolerance and frequent consumption of baked egg is associated with tolerating all forms of egg sooner than those who are not baked egg–tolerant.

AVOIDANCE LIST:

- Albumin (also spelled albumen)
- Egg (dried, powdered, solid, white, yolk)
- Eggnog
- Lysozyme
- Mayonnaise
- Meringue (meringue powder)
- Ovalbumin
- Surimi

Egg is *sometimes* found in:

- Baked goods
- Egg substitutes
- Lecithin
- Macaroni
- Marzipan
- Marshmallows
- Nougat
- Pasta

Though by no means likely, egg can be found in the following:

* Foam or topping on specialty coffee drinks and some bar drinks.
* Most commercially processed cooked pastas (e.g., those used in prepared foods such as soup) contain egg or are processed on equipment shared with egg-containing pastas. Boxed, dry pastas are usually egg-free, but may be processed on equipment that is also used for egg-containing products. Fresh pasta is sometimes egg-free, too.
* Egg wash (used as a "lacquer" to make rolls or sucking candy shiny; on pretzels before they are dipped in salt).

As a Component of Vaccine, Egg Is Safe (With a Qualification)

The MMR vaccine (measles-mumps-rubella) may safely be given to those with egg allergy, including ones with a history of severe, generalized anaphylactic reaction to egg. The recommendation, made by the American Academy of Pediatrics, is based on long-standing scientific evidence that supports one-dose administration as routine.

Flu vaccines usually contain egg protein in small amount. Similar to MMR, flu vaccines in all forms, including the nasal vaccine, have been shown to be safe for egg-allergic individuals, including those with severe reactions including anaphylaxis. As of the fall of 2016, flu vaccines may be given to egg-allergic persons by primary care providers in the office as a single dose, without special precautions. Although rarely given in the United States, yellow fever vaccine also contains egg, and is the only egg-containing vaccine where evaluation is required by a trained specialist before its administration to an egg-allergic individual.

For the Birds

■

Because eggs from duck, turkey, goose, quail, etc., are potentially cross-reactive with hen's egg, they should be avoided.

PEANUTS

Peanuts grow underground, not on trees—as (of course) tree nuts do—and are in fact not part of the nut family but the legume family, which includes beans, peas, lentils, and soybeans.

Interestingly, those who are peanut-allergic are not at greater risk of allergy to another legume than they are to any other food, and legumes do not need to be avoided because of peanut allergy unless the individual has reacted independently to a legume. A small percentage of those who are peanut-allergic may be tree nut–allergic, as well. Approximately 25 to 40 percent of such people are "cosensitized" and test positive to tree nuts; historically, we've urged caution in such cases even if the person has not previously eaten tree nut. If you are (or suspect you might be) such a person, discuss the situation with your allergy provider; where appropriate, a food challenge may be recommended to determine only those allergens that need to be avoided.

AVOIDANCE LIST

- Artificial nuts
- Beer nuts
- Cold-pressed, expelled, or extruded peanut oil
- Goobers
- Ground nuts
- Mandelonas (peanuts soaked in almond flavoring)
- Mixed nuts

- Monkey nuts
- Nut meat
- Nut pieces
- Peanut butter
- Peanut flour
- Peanut protein hydrolysate

Peanut is *sometimes* found in:

- Baked goods (e.g., pastries, cookies)
- Candy (including chocolate candy)
- Chili
- Egg rolls
- Enchilada sauce
- Marzipan
- Mole sauce
- Nougat

Though by no means likely, peanut can be found in the following:

- African, Mexican, Asian (particularly Chinese, Indian, Thai, Vietnamese, and Indonesian) dishes
- Sauces such as chili sauce, hot sauce, pesto, gravy, mole, and salad dressing
- Sweets such as pudding, pies, and hot chocolate
- Pancakes
- Specialty pizzas
- Some vegetarian food products, especially those advertised as meat substitutes
- Foods that contain extruded, cold-pressed or expelled peanut oil, which may contain peanut protein
- Glazes and marinades
- Pet food

Clean Thoroughly

■

According to one study, cleaning with antibacterial gel alone is not sufficient for eliminating traces of peanut from your hands (or body). Cleaning with running water and soap, or commercial wipes, will work. Dishwashing liquid is inadequate on its own to clean away peanut from surfaces; common household spray cleaners and sanitizing wipes will work.

Foods possibly processed on equipment used for peanuts or tree nuts:

- Sunflower seeds
- Alternative nut butters (soy nut butter, sunflower seed butter)

TREE NUTS

Tree nuts are drupaceous fruits from various trees. Their allergens frequently cross-react with tree pollen, as well as peanut. Tree nut allergy is growing at a similar rate to peanut allergy. Only about 10 percent of those diagnosed with tree nut allergy are expected to outgrow the allergy.

It's a Process

■

Food oils (e.g., corn, peanut, soy) can range from mildly to highly allergenic. It largely depends on how much of the food protein was eliminated during processing. Highly refined peanut oil does not contain peanut protein and is safe for consumption by most people. Avoid cold-pressed, fresher, and smaller-batched peanut oils that may contain some degree of peanut protein.

> ## Peanut Is Not a Nut? Well, Neither Are These.
> ▣
>
> Butternut squash
> Nutmeg
> Water chestnut

Numerous establishments—for example, bakeries, ice cream parlors, and certain ethnic restaurants (e.g., Chinese, African, Indian, Thai, and Vietnamese)—commonly include nuts in a range of dishes, making cross-contact possible. If you're allergic to tree nuts, this potentially heightens your exposure risk, even if you order and consume dishes described as tree nut–free.

Identifying problematic nuts may be difficult, for kids and adults both. In one study, peanut was the most easily identified nut, unsurprisingly; filbert (hazelnut), the least. An improved ability to identify nuts would help, particularly since peanuts and tree nuts are the leading cause of food-related anaphylaxis.

The FDA has a rather expanded list of what they consider a tree nut. Many allergists would not agree with some of their designations; some of these "nuts" are more fleshy fruits than hard nuts, and there have been very few reported reactions to them. But their presence on the list may raise anxiety and create unnecessary avoidance, rather than provide protection against a likely allergen. Below, I've designated these "nuts" with an asterisk (*). Still, if you are allergic to tree nuts, please first discuss with your allergist or health care provider the risks and benefits of consuming the starred foods before doing so.

AVOIDANCE LIST
- Almond
- Artificial nuts
- Brazil nut
- Beechnut*

- Butternut*
- Cashew (pink peppercorn—known as Brazilian pepper—rose pepper, Christmasberry, and others may pose a risk to those allergic to cashew in very rare circumstances)
- Chestnut
- Chinquapin nut*
- Coconut (allergic reaction to coconut is very rare and most tree nut allergic individuals safely eat it; still, as stated earlier, this should be discussed with your allergist)
- Filbert/hazelnut
- Gianduja (a chocolate-nut mixture)
- Ginkgo nut*
- Hazelnut
- Hickory nut*
- Lychee nut*
- Macadamia nut (technically a seed, but often lumped into the tree nut category)
- Marzipan/almond paste
- Nangai nut*
- Natural nut extract (e.g., almond, walnut)
- Nut butters (e.g., cashew butter)
- Nut meal
- Nut meat
- Nut milk (e.g., almond milk, cashew milk)
- Nut paste (e.g., almond paste)
- Nut pieces
- Pecan
- Pesto (may contain walnut, pine nut, or both, depending on the recipe)
- Pili nut
- Pine nut (technically a seed, but often lumped in with tree nuts; also referred to as Indian, pignola, pignolia, pignon, piñon, and pinyon nut)
- Pistachio

- Praline
- Shea nut*
- Walnut

Tree nut is *sometimes* found in:

- (Black) walnut hull extract (flavoring)
- Natural nut extracts, such as pure almond extract (imitation/ artificially flavored extracts are generally safe)
- Nut distillates/alcoholic extracts
- Nut oils (e.g., walnut oil, almond oil; they may be used in lotions, soaps, and hair care products; in lotions, nut oil is unlikely to cause a reaction, but it may irritate the skin or allow sensitization through broken-down skin. The risk of these oils in beauty products is unknown and unlikely to cause a reaction, but discuss using these products with your provider first)

Though by no means likely, tree nuts can be found in the following:

- Alcoholic beverages may contain nut flavoring (though this could be artificial flavoring and contain no nut protein)
- Barbecue sauces
- Candy
- Cereal
- Chocolates
- Cold cuts such as mortadella
- Cookies
- Crackers
- Energy bars
- Flavored coffee
- Frozen desserts
- Marinades

FIN FISH

It's estimated that two in five fish-allergic individuals may suffer their first reaction to fin fish as adults, though an appreciable number of children develop this allergy, too. Unlike most other food allergies, allergy to finned fish usually does not resolve over time. Some of those allergic to fish react to more than one type, as the allergenic protein is highly conserved across the various fish species. Fish allergy can induce severe reactions, including anaphylaxis.

While the allergen is generally found in the protein in the fish's flesh, exposure to fish gelatin, composed of fish skin and bones, may also cause a reaction. Fish oil, ostensibly free of protein, may still be tainted by protein in the extraction process, thus posing risk. When fish is cooked, protein can become airborne, making the steam a risk, though this is very rarely reported.

An allergy to finned fish does not mean an allergy to shellfish, which is not from a related food family. These food families are unrelated and have different allergenic proteins.

AVOIDANCE LIST

There are an estimated twenty thousand-plus species of fish. Salmon, tuna, and cod cause the most reactions. A list of those and the other main culprits:

- Anchovy
- Bass
- Catfish
- Cod
- Flounder
- Grouper
- Haddock
- Hake
- Halibut
- Herring

- Mahimahi
- Perch
- Pike
- Pollock
- Salmon
- Scrod
- Sole
- Snapper
- Swordfish
- Tilapia
- Trout
- Tuna

Fish can be found in the following:

- Barbecue sauce
- Bouillabaisse
- Caesar salad and Caesar dressing
- Caponata, a Sicilian eggplant relish
- Imitation or artificial fish or shellfish (e.g., surimi, also known as "sea legs" or "sea sticks")
- Meat loaf
- Worcestershire sauce

Cross-Contact Concern

■

Take extra care at certain ethnic restaurants (e.g., Chinese, African, Indonesian, Thai, and Vietnamese), which use fish and fish ingredients extensively; there may be cross-contact with these and non-fish items. Some Asian restaurants employ fish sauce to flavor the base of non-fish items. Also, cooking utensils and pots/pans/woks may not be cleaned in between uses at these restaurants.

SHELLFISH

It's estimated that three in five shellfish-allergic individuals may suffer their first reaction as adults, though this is a well-known allergen among children, too. Unlike most other food allergies, allergy to shellfish usually does not resolve over time. Of the two types of shellfish—crustacean (soft-shelled creatures such as shrimp, crab, and lobster) and mollusks (hard-shelled creatures such as clams, mussels, oysters, and scallops)—the former are associated with more frequent reactions, though allergy to either can occur. Allergy to one shellfish group family does not automatically mean allergy to the other. Still, since most shellfish-allergic individuals may react to more than one type, it's probably wise to avoid this food family entirely.

Avoid touching shellfish. When shellfish is cooked, the protein can become airborne, making the steam a risk, though this is exceptionally rare.

You may also be wise to avoid seafood restaurants because a non-seafood item that you order may cross-contact with seafood.

AVOIDANCE LIST

The bulk of shellfish allergies are triggered by shrimp, crab, and lobster.

- Barnacle
- Crab
- Crawfish (crawdad, crayfish, écrevisse)
- Krill
- Lobster (langouste, langoustine, Moreton bay bugs, scampi, tomalley)
- Prawns
- Shrimp (crevette, scampi)

The Food Allergen Labeling and Consumer Protection Act (FAL-CPA) does not consider mollusks a major allergen group, thus their inclusion in a product may not be labeled or labeled fully. Yet you may need to avoid the following:

- Abalone
- Clams (cherrystone, geoduck, littleneck, pismo, quahog)
- Cockle
- Cuttlefish (often a component of paella)
- Limpet (lapas, opihi)
- Mussels
- Octopus
- Oysters
- Periwinkle
- Scallops
- Sea cucumber
- Sea urchin
- Snails (escargot)
- Squid (calamari)
- Whelk (turban shell)

Though by no means likely, shellfish can be found in the following:

- Bouillabaisse
- Cuttlefish ink
- Glucosamine
- Fish stock
- Seafood flavoring (e.g., crab or clam extract)
- Surimi

WHEAT

One of the most common food allergies in children, wheat allergy, is often outgrown in childhood—in one study, more than half of kids had outgrown it by age eight. Given that wheat is our leading grain product, what might make up a wheat-free diet? Alternate grains include amaranth, barley, corn, oat, quinoa, rice, rye, and tapioca. When baking, you might wish to combine wheat-free flours because they provide superior texture to using only one grain. One popular blend is made of flours from rice, potato starch, and tapioca.

Approximately one in five wheat-allergic children may have tolerance issues with other grains, too. Wheat often cross-reacts on allergy tests with certain species of grass and other grains; in other words, tests frequently come up positive, yet the individuals do not experience an allergic reaction after ingesting the food. The true implications of a positive test may be determined by a supervised food challenge.

Consult with your doctor about the safety of foods containing barley, oats, or rye—these are generally tolerated in wheat allergy, but may pose a risk in wheat-induced FPIES, a delayed gastrointestinal reaction to certain foods seen in infants to very young children. Symptoms include profuse vomiting, diarrhea, and associated dehydration.

AVOIDANCE LIST

- Bread crumbs
- Bulgur
- Cereal extract
- Club wheat
- Couscous
- Cracker meal
- Durum
- Einkorn
- Emmer
- Farina
- Flour (all-purpose, bread, cake, durum, enriched, graham, high-gluten, high-protein, instant, pastry, self-rising, soft wheat, steel ground, stone ground, whole wheat)
- Hydrolyzed wheat protein
- Kamut
- Matzoh, matzoh meal (also spelled as matzo, matzah, or matza)

What's Wheat Allergy, What's Celiac Disease, What's Gluten Intolerance?

If you've got wheat allergy, it works like this: Eating wheat exposes you to the protein that triggers your immune system to overreact. Symptoms range from mild (hives, rash, itching, swelling) to severe (wheezing, trouble breathing, loss of consciousness) to potentially life-threatening.

Celiac disease is a genetic autoimmune disorder, the most common of its kind, that compromises the body's ability to digest gluten, a protein in barley, rye, and wheat. The immune system essentially attacks its own tissue: Certain antibodies are produced against various gluten proteins, obstructing the intestines' ability to properly absorb key nutrients. If left untreated, celiac disease can lead to medical difficulties including intestinal damage, malnutrition, potential malignancy, other autoimmune conditions, osteoporosis, and infertility. The good news? It's the one autoimmune disorder whose trigger is clear, and thus largely avoidable. If you have celiac disease and you're on a gluten-free diet, you can truly be as symptom-free and healthy as if you did not have the disease. Celiac disease has clear genetic factors; the HLA gene test may help confirm diagnosis. But it's important to understand that gluten-mediated enteropathy (another name for celiac disease) is clinically distinct from IgE-mediated wheat allergy, though both necessitate strict wheat avoidance.

Gluten intolerance is also known as non-celiac gluten sensitivity but sometimes used as an umbrella term for that, celiac disease, and wheat allergy. It is not all three. Gluten intolerance is not thought to be immune-mediated. When exposed to wheat, a gluten-intolerant individual can experience gastrointestinal tract problems or other symptoms, but the mechanism producing these are unclear. There is no available test to confirm a diagnosis of gluten intolerance. (There is a test for lactose intolerance and fructose intolerance.)

- Pasta
- Seitan
- Semolina
- Spelt
- Sprouted wheat
- Triticale
- Vital wheat gluten
- Wheat (bran, durum, germ, gluten, grass, malt, sprouts, starch)
- Wheat bran hydrolysate
- Wheat germ oil
- Wheat grass
- Wheat protein isolate
- Whole wheat berries

Wheat is *sometimes* found in:

- Beer
- Cider
- Glucose syrup
- Soy sauce
- Starch (gelatinized starch, modified starch, modified food starch, vegetable starch)
- Surimi

Though by no means likely, wheat can be found in the following:

- Ale
- Baked products
- Baking mixes
- Batter-fried foods
- Breaded foods
- Breakfast cereals
- Candy
- Crackers

In-Grained

■

It's been my experience that a notable percentage of those with food-induced exercise allergy have wheat, in any form or food, as a trigger. It's hypothesized that a particular protein in wheat, one of several food allergens thought to be pivotal in this condition, when activated by exertion, could be the cause, and it can occur with wheat ingestion several hours before or even after exercise, making diagnosis and avoidance difficult. Here's one example that I encountered: Almost every time my patient Brad hit the gym, usually to run on the treadmill, he was forced to curtail his workout because he got overly red and hot, and developed a rash over much of his upper body. Fortunately, these symptoms were not accompanied by respiratory complications such as trouble breathing or swallowing. In Brad's case, it was limited to his skin, and he immediately knew to stop exercising. Upon testing, we identified a likely sensitivity to wheat; another test confirmed allergy to it. And it turned out that, before his "power workouts," he would almost always eat a cereal power bar that contained wheat. Brad responded well to the simple recommendation to refrain from eating, particularly anything containing wheat, for at least four to six hours before exercise, and of course to carry with him an epinephrine auto-injector. Prophylaxis is the key: We strive to prevent a recurrence.

- Hot dogs
- Ice cream (some brands)
- Imitation crabmeat (some types)
- Marinara sauce
- Play dough
- Potato chips
- Processed meats
- Rice cakes

> ## Bucking the Trend
>
> ■
>
> Wheat and buckwheat are not related. However, buckwheat is an emerging allergen in both the United States and Japan.

- Salad dressings
- Sauces
- Soups
- Turkey patties

SOY

Soybean allergy is one of the more common food allergies, particularly in babies and children. Soy allergy is often outgrown in childhood, and studies show that most children outgrow it by age ten.

Reaction to soy can be severe. As with those allergic to peanuts—which, like soy, is a legume—those allergic to soy are not at greater risk for allergy to another legume than they are to any other food. It used to be that doctors recommended that their peanut-allergic patients avoid soy, too, but their concern now appears unwarranted, and such caution unnecessary.

Soybeans alone generally do not constitute a major portion of one's diet. However, soy is a component in many foods and dishes, so to maintain a proper diet, it's important to replace the lost nutrients in some form. Many labels note the inclusion of soy in the form of soy lecithin. This is not a soy protein–containing form and is generally (if not universally) tolerated by soy-allergic individuals. When such a person reads "contains soy" on a label and eschews the product, it may be unnecessary.

Soy oil tends to be highly refined and does not contain appreciable soy protein, and is likely safe, too.

AVOIDANCE LIST
- Edamame
- Miso
- Natto
- Shoyu
- Soy (soy albumin, soy cheese, soy fiber, soy flour, soy grits, soy ice cream, soy milk, soy nuts, soy sprouts, soy yogurt)
- Soya
- Soybean (curd, granules)
- Soy protein (concentrate, hydrolyzed, isolate)
- Soy sauce (may also contain wheat)
- Tamari
- Tempeh
- Textured vegetable protein (TVP)
- Tofu

Soy is *sometimes* found in:

- Asian cuisine
- Vegetable broth
- Vegetable gum
- Vegetable starch

Though by no means likely, soy (soybeans and soy products) can be found in the following:

- Baked goods
- Canned broths and soups
- Canned tuna and meat
- Cereals

The Height of Refinement

■

Highly refined soybean oil is not labeled as an allergen. Research shows that for most soy-allergic individuals, it's safe to eat soybean oil that is highly refined—as opposed to soybean oil that is "cold-pressed," "extruded," or "expeller-pressed."

- Cookies
- Crackers
- High-protein energy bars and snacks
- Infant formulas
- Low-fat peanut butter
- Processed meats
- Sauces

Sesame: The 9th of the Big 8

■

Hundreds of thousands of Americans are allergic to sesame. Sesame oil contains sesame protein; data suggest that anaphylaxis can occur with exposure to sesame oil. As we have access to, and eat more, "exotic" foods from other cultures, we become exposed to ingredients that are less common in the United States. The Food Labeling Modernization Act of 2015 would potentially add sesame to the list of major food allergens that require clear, specific disclosure on labels, though changes to FALCPA may be difficult to initiate. In Canada, sesame is treated as a major allergen, and the Canadian Food Inspection Agency (CFIA) enforces certain labeling requirements because of it.

Overcooked

An allergist colleague told me about a friend who, after hosting a Fourth of July cookout, wound up in the local ER covered with hives; a blood test helped to determine that he had alpha gal–related red meat allergy associated with the bite from a Lone Star tick.

Those affected by this condition develop an antibody to the sugar, alpha gal, found in pork, lamb, and beef. If you're bitten by a Lone Star tick, an allergic reaction may occur four hours or more after you've eaten red meat. Few are familiar with this food allergy, but for the small number of patients I've heard of who've endured it, it's highly unpleasant.

My colleague advised his patient that he could keep grilling—but with precautions to minimize and hopefully eliminate the potential for cross-contact with red meat. There's always veggie burgers, fish, and chicken.

How Do Little Kids Let Us Know They're Experiencing Food Allergy?

Being the parent or caregiver of a food-allergic child is an experience filled with fear and anxiety. Will it happen? Will it happen again? When will it happen? Who will be around when it happens? Will my child know what to do? Will she let those around her know, in a timely manner?

Many food-allergic kids are too young or developmentally immature to express themselves with perfect clarity. They will try to communicate that they are experiencing abdominal pain, itchiness, or other bodily changes that represent early signs of a serious allergic reaction—or they may express their discomfort differently and less specifically. Be attentive to statements like these:

It feels like something is poking my tongue.
My tongue (or mouth) is tingling (or burning).
My tongue (or mouth) itches.
My tongue feels like there is hair on it.
My mouth feels funny.
There's a frog in my throat; there's something stuck in my throat.
My tongue feels full (or heavy).
My lips feel tight.
It feels like there are bugs in there (to describe itchy ears).
It (my throat) feels thick.
It feels like a bump is on the back of my tongue (throat).[1]

Aside from the potential physiological threat that weighs on your child and you, there's the mental/psychological one: How do you help your child to have a normal sense of herself? You're not alone in the fear and stress you feel, of course: She feels it, too, especially if she's already had a life-threatening reaction. Does the fear limit her social life, and what she does on a day-to-day basis? Does she feel isolated, or as if she's burdening those around her? Is she teased, bullied or harassed about her food allergy by peers? It's not unusual for such kids to be burdened with anxiety over their condition.

---

1. Statements children may make: © 2016, Food Allergy Research & Education. Adapted and used with permission.

Be Prepared, Here and There

If you have a food allergy:

1. Wear medical identification jewelry.
2. When eating outside the home, carry a food allergy card explaining your allergy.
3. Carry two epinephrine auto-injectors.
4. Make sure friends you're dining with—and the chef or restaurant manager, too—know of your allergy and how to use your auto-injector. A companion, or someone present, should know beforehand the steps to take if something happens.
5. Have safe snacks with you.

If you're on the road or out of the country:

1. For upcoming weddings, business conferences, and other events where meals are being prepared, contact the organizer or caterer to get details.
2. Carry translation cards that spell out your allergy, what happens if you encounter the allergen, and what treatment you require. Show it to your host, waiter, and anyone involved with providing you food. If even trace allergen amounts are potentially serious, make sure it's indicated. Selectwisely.com and allergytranslation.com create cards in many languages.
3. The food labeling in other countries is not always like ours. How does theirs work? How accurate is it? Not all countries use a form of the phrase "may contain." Some countries use numeric codes.
4. Does your lodging have a kitchen you can use? The ability to prepare your own meals may make your vacation or business trip much less stressful.

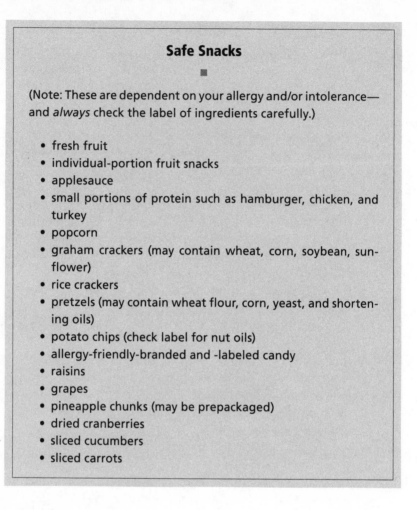

Safe Snacks

■

(Note: These are dependent on your allergy and/or intolerance—and *always* check the label of ingredients carefully.)

- fresh fruit
- individual-portion fruit snacks
- applesauce
- small portions of protein such as hamburger, chicken, and turkey
- popcorn
- graham crackers (may contain wheat, corn, soybean, sunflower)
- rice crackers
- pretzels (may contain wheat flour, corn, yeast, and shortening oils)
- potato chips (check label for nut oils)
- allergy-friendly-branded and -labeled candy
- raisins
- grapes
- pineapple chunks (may be prepackaged)
- dried cranberries
- sliced cucumbers
- sliced carrots

Oral Allergy Syndrome and Cross-Reactivity

Many of my patients report itching and/or mild swelling of the mouth and throat immediately following their eating of certain uncooked fruits (including nuts) or raw vegetables. The symptoms result from contact in the oropharynx (the mid-part of the throat behind the mouth). What is this, and why does it happen?

Oral allergy syndrome (OAS), also known as pollen-food syndrome, is estimated to be the most prevalent "food allergy" among adults, though it's technically not a food allergy but rather a pollen allergy that cross-reacts with certain foods (if that makes sense). It's believed to affect upward of 5 percent of the population, and a much higher percentage among pollen-sensitive allergic individuals. Anecdotally, it appears that the rate of OAS has increased, in large part because the rate of pollen allergy has also increased over the last couple decades.

Why would the latter jump influence the former? Because of a phenomenon known as cross-reactivity. An antibody reaction is triggered not merely to one food allergen but to another, similar allergen—in this case, pollen. (By similar, I mean that when you eat that particular food, the immune system recognizes proteins in it similar to those in pollen that it's already guarding against/reacting to.) OAS is the result of an existing allergy to one of the varieties of pollen (tree, weed, less so with grass) in combination with exposure to a particular uncooked plant food, or plant food from a particular food family. (Non-plant foods— e.g., egg, milk, shellfish—are not a factor in OAS.) While children may experience OAS, it's more common in adults largely because it requires you first to have developed pollen allergy, which for many people takes repeated exposure and is likelier to occur as one ages. This combination—where the existence of two conditions leads to a reaction—is cross-reactivity. (Note that not all OAS sufferers have obvious hay fever or seasonal allergy symptoms.)

OAS symptoms generally include mild itching or tingling in the mouth and/or mild swelling in the mouth and throat. Blisters may occur, though rarely by themselves. Symptoms develop while or shortly after (within five to ten minutes of) ingestion of the culprit fruit, vegetable, or nut, and resolve fairly quickly. More serious symptoms, including anaphylaxis, are fairly uncommon, affecting from 2 to 10 percent of OAS individuals; in the event of anaphylaxis, it's generally restricted to GI symptoms (vomiting).

Severity of the OAS reaction may be influenced by numerous factors: the food's level of ripeness/freshness, your current level of antibod-

Heat Labile vs. Heat Stable

■

Some foods, such as tree nut, fish, shellfish and peanut, are heat stable: They maintain their disruptive power whether they're raw or cooked; that is, the heat from cooking does not degrade the allergenicity of the proteins. Other foods, such as certain egg and milk proteins, apple and other fruits, and vegetables, are heat labile, and they are allergenic in their raw form but less so or not at all in their cooked form (or with milk and egg, yes in their low/pan-heated forms but maybe no in their extensively heated forms), and thus may not cause the expected allergic symptoms.

ies, stomach acidity, use of NSAIDs or other medication, even recent exercise. For some, the skin/peel of the food is the problem; for others, it's the pulp/flesh; for others, it doesn't matter which.

Some cross-reactive combinations are likelier than others to trigger severe reaction. There may be sensitivity to a particular pollen and a particular food, or perhaps to two foods—e.g., mugwort-mustard syndrome. A type of OAS is latex-fruit, or latex-food, syndrome. As many as half of those allergic to natural rubber latex have exhibited hypersensitivity to some plant foods, especially fresh fruits and related foods like avocado, banana, bell pepper, chestnut, kiwi, peach, tomato, and white potato. In one study, a patient who was ultimately determined to have celery-mugwort-birch-spice syndrome suffered anaphylaxis after the stress of exercise was added.

OAS is usually a lifelong condition, though you may improve it through immunotherapy for pollen allergy; the FDA has approved some sublingual immunotherapy tablets for ragweed and grass pollen because the tablets have been shown to reduce symptoms. However, this is effective for only some sufferers.

At times, what appears to be OAS may not be that at all. Other possible conditions:

Fuzzy Fruits

Throughout Europe, both in the north and also the Mediterranean, peach is among the most common causes of food allergy. Kiwi allergy is also prevalent in Europe: One study found that nearly half of food-allergic individuals in Sweden and Denmark reacted to kiwi; another study demonstrated that 4 percent of allergic kids tested positive for the fruit (though that does not necessarily mean they can't eat it). Young kids are much likelier than adults to react after their first exposure to kiwi, and to experience serious symptoms.

This all may be due to the proximity and prevalence of birch.

Recently, a patient of mine noticed an itchy sensation in her throat, and irritation that caused a short coughing attack and near gagging. She already had pronounced seasonal springtime allergies. In-office skin testing revealed a significant positive result to birch tree pollen. It turned out that, not long before the attack, she had eaten fruit salad, with kiwi generously mixed in.

Contact urticaria—certain foods (e.g., citrus fruit, garlic, berries, tomato sauce) cause local irritation of the lips and the skin around the mouth. Similarly, irritation by foods that are spicy, tart, or gritty (e.g., pineapple) cause irritation to the mouth, tongue, or throat.

Perioral dermatitis or oral contact dermatitis—caused by contact with mango or cashews, or with cosmetic products, in those vulnerable to poison ivy.

Gastroesophageal reflux disease (GERD)—a digestive disorder whose symptoms, including heartburn that frequently feels higher up the neck and throat, are often exacerbated after eating.

Eosinophilic esophagitis (EoE)—you may have the feeling that food is lodged in the throat, due to swelling or inflammation of the esophagus. EoE can cause gagging, food impaction and choking, nausea, vomiting, abdominal pain; in certain individuals, it can lead to weight loss.

Burning mouth syndrome—reported mostly by women middle-aged or older; burning (as opposed to itching) feeling in and around the oral cavity.

While OAS is best managed by avoiding any fruits and vegetables that cause a reaction, in most cases you may need only to avoid those foods in their raw form. Cooking—the addition of heat—tends to break down the proteins, rendering them harmless. (Digestion breaks down the proteins as well.) To give one example, whereas eating a raw apple may cause itching, eating apple pie or applesauce, or drinking pasteurized apple juice, may cause no harm. Note, however, that this is *not* true of peanuts and tree nuts: In fact, roasting nuts can make them *more* allergenic and able to trigger OAS in those who are susceptible.

When testing for OAS, false readings, both positive and negative, are not uncommon. Fresh food testing using a prick-to-prick method (prick the food item, then gently prick the patient's skin) may be recommended.

Recurrent Swallowing and Choking

■

Choking may occur from mechanical obstruction that traps food as it goes down the food pipe, or esophagus, creating the choking risk. This condition is generally found in those who already suffer from acid reflux, heartburn, and the like. In many cases, it is suspected to be an allergic reaction to a food, but this is not always the case, and for many people with eosinophilic esophagitis (EoE), there may not be a dietary component. A gastroenterologist can confirm EoE, an increasingly prevalent condition. I myself am seeing it more and more; I'd estimate it's three times as prevalent in my own practice as it once was. Fortunately, it's a malady that, for the most part, can be managed successfully. There needs to be greater awareness of this condition by all of us, especially when choking and/or food impaction can present as a medical emergency.

Medications to control acid reflux often provide relief to that and an end to the choking, as well. If food allergy *is* present, testing may provide clues.

CROSS-REACTIVITY: WHAT GOES WITH WHAT

Allergy trigger	Cross-reactors

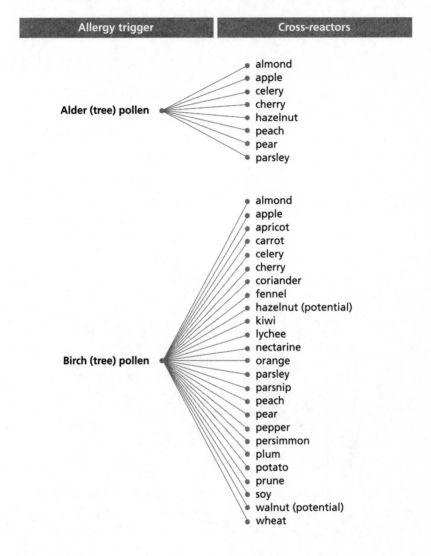

Alder (tree) pollen
- almond
- apple
- celery
- cherry
- hazelnut
- peach
- pear
- parsley

Birch (tree) pollen
- almond
- apple
- apricot
- carrot
- celery
- cherry
- coriander
- fennel
- hazelnut (potential)
- kiwi
- lychee
- nectarine
- orange
- parsley
- parsnip
- peach
- pear
- pepper
- persimmon
- plum
- potato
- prune
- soy
- walnut (potential)
- wheat

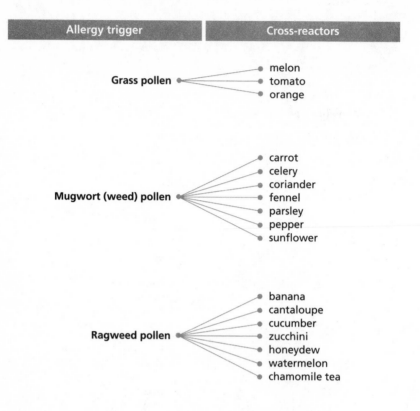

Allergy trigger	Cross-reactors
Grass pollen	melon tomato orange
Mugwort (weed) pollen	carrot celery coriander fennel parsley pepper sunflower
Ragweed pollen	banana cantaloupe cucumber zucchini honeydew watermelon chamomile tea

Labeling

The Food Allergen Labeling and Consumer Protection Act (FALCPA) went into effect at the start of 2006, requiring US food manufacturers to list the ingredients of prepared foods; to use plain language to disclose the presence, or possible presence, of any of the eight common food allergens—egg, milk, peanut, tree nuts, fish, crustacean shellfish, wheat, and soy; and to update label requirements for food products overseen by the Food and Drug Administration (FDA). These FDA-regulated foods include those sold at food-service and retail establishments; foods in vending machines; packaged foods; diet supplements and vitamins; infant formula and foods; and more. In 2013, the FDA ruled that items labeled "gluten-free" must satisfy a defined standard for gluten content.

What does FALCPA *not* cover? Fresh fruits and vegetables in their natural state; highly refined oil that comes from one of the Big 8 allergen foods; any ingredient derived from such highly refined oil; prescription and OTC drugs; cosmetics, shampoo, mouthwash, toothpaste, shaving cream, and other personal care products; any USDA-regulated food "product" (e.g., meat, poultry, some egg products); any Alcohol, Tobacco Tax and Trade Bureau–regulated product, such as beer, spirits, and other alcoholic drinks and tobacco products; restaurant foods, including fast food; food from vendors and street fairs/festivals; pet foods; and more. Allergens such as seeds or mollusk shellfish are, similarly, not labeled.

If you or your loved one is food-allergic, no doubt you already read labels carefully. They provide a list not just of major ingredients but, in

"May Contain . . ."

FALCPA states that the eight major allergens must be labeled in simple terms. It may be done in the ingredients list or in a separate allergen statement. However, FALCPA does not enforce "advisory" or "precautionary" labeling. A phrase such as "may contain" is therefore employed voluntarily. It does not project specific risks—and indeed it's impossible to say what result will occur for the food-allergic who use that product. Some research shows that such precautionary labeling usually implies very low levels of contamination (in parts per million, which would represent roughly a soda-bottle's worth of water in a 50-meter Olympic-size pool), which would likely be tolerated by even very sensitive individuals. There are multiple emerging data on threshold levels but no clear statement yet on the safety of such precautionary labeling.

the case of the Big 8, the specific type (e.g., almond, walnut; bass, floun-der); additives or by-products; and (for many products) whether the food was produced in a facility that processes other potential allergens, such as nuts. Just because you've read the label on a particular food product, know that it can change abruptly: Manufacturers often alter ingredients.

Foods made locally may not always comply with FALCPA stan-dards. (Then again, they may.)

Spices

It's exceptionally rare, and estimated that under 1 percent of the popula-tion succumbs to a variety of reactions after ingesting spices. The most allergy-provoking spice families are Apiaceae, which includes caraway, fennel, celery, coriander, and dill, and Liliaceae, which includes chive, shallot, garlic, onion, and saffron. A possible spice-allergic individual may have an associated pollen allergy, and for many in this situation, the allergy manifests as skin-contact irritation.

The level of allergenicity is influenced by the spice itself, as well as its processing (or lack of processing): Is it raw, roasted, boiled, toasted, fried? Interestingly, the addition of heat may, depending on conditions, either decrease *or* increase a spice's allergenicity.

Spices are prevalent components in many non-foods: peppermint and cinnamon oil are used to flavor alcoholic beverages, toothpaste and dental products; cloves and oil of cinnamon are used in massage oil. Cosmetics, fragrances, and body oils may contain allspice, anise, balsam of Peru, caraway, cinnamon, cloves, curry, ginger, star anise, sesame seed, vanilla, or rosemary. Because of the presence of spices in cosmet-ics, women are likelier than men to develop spice allergy, most notably skin allergy/allergic contact dermatitis.

American Pastime

■

A patient came in, pretty sure that his recent allergic reaction was triggered by a hot dog he ate at a baseball game. I investigated the hot dog possibility, and also turned my attention to the condiments he used—and he tested positive to mustard (seed and powder). He happily returned to eating hot dogs at baseball games, this time substituting relish and/or ketchup for his (admittedly beloved) mustard.

Food Additives

There are eight major food allergens; there also happen to be eight major food additives, among the thousands (both natural and artificial) that exist, that may cause adverse reactions. Additive and dye reactions are often alleged but, fortunately, rarely substantiated. The reactions caused are very different from those triggered by the food allergens described previously; these do not involve IgE. Relatively few people are affected, and the symptoms, which vary by additive, do not last more than a day; it's usually much less than that. The additives or additive families that have been investigated include:

- *Sulfites.* Used to preserve freshness; some sulfites are natural, most are artificial.
- *Aspartame (e.g., Nutrasweet).* Zero-calorie sweetener used in beverages and food.
- *Parabens.* Preservative in food, medication, shampoos, sunscreen, and more.
- *Tartrazine.* Yellow dye used in beverages, candy, cheese, hot dogs, salad dressing, and more.
- *Monosodium glutamate, glutamic acid (MSG).* Flavor enhancer in food, including packaged meat.

- *Nitrates and nitrites.* Preserves food, prevents botulism contamination, enhances flavor, colors food. Used in hot dogs, salami, other meats, and fish.
- *Butylated hydroxytoluene (BHT) and butylated hydroxyanisole (BHA).* Preservatives in breakfast cereal, other grain products.
- *Benzoates.* Preservatives in cake, cereal, candy, salad dressing, and more.

The reactions to additives are not considered allergic but rather pharmacological (that is, most everyone is affected—such as with the stimulant effect of caffeine) or idiopathic (an uncommon reaction that's not understood, with no clear mechanism). Those who react to one additive are unlikely to react to another that's chemically unrelated.

Diagnosis

Given the dizzying, often elusive array of foods and food components that can trigger a reaction, and the added fact that many reactions are not allergic in nature and may be the result of a different food-related condition altogether, I strongly recommend that if you suspect an allergy-like situation with you or your child, go see an allergist. Years of training have given us the experience at determining which tests, if any, are needed, how to interpret results, and managing next steps. I've seen multiple situations where a patient comes in having been given the wrong test, which led her down an unwarranted path. Not only does this mean a delay in the right treatment, it also means that she (a) needlessly deprived herself of a certain food, and the nutrients to be derived from it (not to mention the pleasure of eating it), and (b) unnecessarily eliminated a food from her diet that she was not allergic to, and when she reintroduced it to her diet after years of abstaining, it triggered an overreaction!

We have numerous tools and ever-expanding knowledge to help diagnose whether one has food allergy, OAS, or something else. Diagnostic testing usually includes these components:

- The patient's general medical history and recent symptoms, and *suspected* food triggers; for example, *Are the symptoms localized around the mouth and in the throat? In other parts of the body? Is there evidence of symptoms of pollen allergy?* It's important to query her about all kinds of foods she may have eaten; often, the patient doesn't volunteer unusual reactions to foods she eats infrequently unless it's brought up.
- A physical exam.
- One or more tests to pinpoint the food allergy, including:

Skin Prick Test (SPT): This is the number one method for assessing food allergy. I place a drop of solution containing an allergen on the patient's forearm (the back is an alternate site). The skin is then gently pricked with a skin test device. (It's truly not painful.) Within about fifteen minutes, there will be resolution: either no reaction or a wheal of some size (it may look like a mosquito bite) indicating recognition of IgE against that item. The larger the wheal/bump, the greater the likelihood of the patient's having a sensitivity to that allergen. Keep in mind that just because you have a positive wheal, it does not always imply that you will react to the particular food allergen that was tested. In addition, your history will help the allergist to properly interpret your test results and create a plan of action. The test's predictive value for negative readings is very good (90 to 95 percent accurate when no IgE antibody is detected).

Food skin prick testing uses commercial food extracts of milk, peanut, almond, walnut, apple, banana, carrot, wheat, soy, egg, etc., rather than raw food.

When testing fresh fruits and vegetables particularly for evaluation of OAS, I might test the food with a method called prick-to-prick testing. A skin tester pricks into the food, then pricks to the skin. It can be a helpful method in certain patients (though sometimes this method can irritate the skin).

As always, there is great variability, depending on the type of food and the symptoms an individual presents with. Still, this method can be helpful in differentiated food allergy and OAS.

Trial Elimination Diet: If I think my patient is dealing with a food allergy, but has no inkling what it could be, I may start cautiously eliminating the suspected food from her diet. I make very specific choices about the food I think is possibly responsible, then monitor any cessation of symptoms. I don't want to eliminate multiple foods at once because (a) it complicates accurate monitoring of symptoms (and their cessation), and (b) it makes life more difficult for you or (when it's a child being tested) your family to have several foods cut out at once. An allergist can help you determine appropriate testing depending on your history. If there is resolution of symptoms with a dietary elimination, then we may have moved closer to identifying the culprit. In some instances, controlled reintroduction of a food is performed, to document that it retriggered the symptoms. Once the culprit is identified, we can reintroduce the eliminated foods that were not causing the problem. The diet may last for days to possibly weeks.

The test may not be conclusive, and I must be wary of subjective reports of improvement. If symptoms return right after we have reintroduced tree nuts (for example), then we have a higher degree of certainty that tree nuts were triggering the symptoms. But it takes some skill in interpreting results. If the trial elimination diet is not conclusive, I may move to the next test for confirmation.

Oral Food Challenge (OFC). It sounds a bit like a reality television show, and the premise is simple: You eat foods commonly suspected of causing allergy—e.g., fish, shellfish, sesame, peanut—under a physician's observation. The upside? It's extremely accurate in identifying allergy. The downside? It can trigger the potentially severe reaction it's trying to uncover—though, as stated, this procedure should be administered under experienced medical supervision only. Because most challenges involve gradually increasing amounts of food, severe reactions are uncommon, and the procedure is halted at the initial emergence of symptoms.

An oral food challenge can help to confirm a diagnosis of food allergy, as well as to determine whether a child or adult has outgrown the food allergy and may thus safely eat the food.

One conclusion reached: Families who underwent an oral food challenge had better quality of life than those who continued avoiding certain suspected food allergens, and never took the challenge—*regardless of the challenge's success!*

Blood Test. In general, this is considered less sensitive than prick skin testing. It measures your level of food allergen–specific IgE antibodies. If the result is negative, then you have a very low likelihood of being allergic to it. A positive result, however, is only mildly helpful: You may react to that food . . . and you may not.

Remember: Allergy is not truly diagnosed by a test. To be allergic, you must have a history of eating a food that causes symptoms. Still, the blood test, as well as the skin tests, can help you to better understand what you may be sensitized (and potentially allergic) to—as well as which allergies may, happily, be a thing of your past.

Food Allergy Resources

Among the great allergy resources out there, a few in particular that have been very helpful and educational to me, my team, and my patients: Food Allergy Research and Education (FARE); Kids with Food Allergies Foundation, acaai.org, and aaaai.org.

Chapter 9

Allergic and Non-Allergic Reactions to Drugs

Often, a patient comes to my office after having been prescribed medication that may have worsened the original problem or created a new one. We'll work backward, using our sleuthing skills to deduce the likely culprit medicine. There are ways to help determine which medicine is more probably to be responsible for a reaction, be it aspirin or an NSAID like ibuprofen or any number of commonly prescribed medications.

The good news about true drug allergy is that it affects only 5 to 10 percent of the population and, more important, there is a wide array of approved, alternative medications. However, the diagnosis of drug allergy can still be challenging, requiring a practitioner experienced in diagnosis and management. What are the main types of drug reactions? What should you know so that you're properly informed about their condition?

A drug allergy is a particular immune response—really, a "hypersensitivity"—to a drug. Drug allergy reactions are largely unpredictable, and may lead to serious, even life-threatening, situations that may require hospitalization and certainly timely therapy. Drug allergy may be caused by any medication—prescription, OTC, herbal, liquid, pill, or injectable form.

The other major category of drug reaction is a predictable adverse reaction. It does not involve the immune system reacting. It is simply a side effect of the drug and, as such, more predictable. In most cases—more than three in four, it's estimated—the bad reaction to a drug is not an allergy or hypersensitivity but an adverse reaction/side effect.

Prescribing or recommending any drug is a carefully weighed decision. A recent study found that when a family of antibiotic drugs called fluoroquinolones was used to treat acute sinusitis, acute bronchitis, and other infections, the serious adverse effects, for the most part, outweighed the benefits. (I can hardly quibble with the findings: One side effect was tendon rupture.)

Still, our lives have been made immeasurably better by so many of these medications, and we're not going to stop using them. Instead, we should be prepared for the possibility that, on occasion, things don't go exactly as we'd hoped with our medications.

MORE COMMON ADVERSE DRUG REACTIONS
(80 PERCENT OF ALL ADRS)

- Predictable, can occur in anyone
- Drug overdose
- Drug interactions—may result in harmful effects
- Drug-to-drug side effects—e.g., diarrhea from antibiotics, gastritis due to NSAIDs (ibuprofen, etc.), hair loss and vomiting due to cancer drugs

LESS COMMON ADVERSE DRUG REACTIONS
(15-20 PERCENT OF ALL ADRS)

- Unpredictable, prior exposure is very likely
- Drug allergy or hypersensitivity (e.g., anaphylaxis after penicillin)
- Intolerance—e.g., ringing of ears (tinnitus) after taking aspirin
- Non-immune—e.g., contrast dyes used in diagnostic X-rays (can premedicate)
- Symptoms vary by severity (both immediate and delayed)—e.g., skin reactions such as rash, hives, flushed skin, swelling of the

skin (angioedema); throat tightness, trouble breathing, wheezing; dizziness and/or a drop in blood pressure; ulcers in the lining of the mouth and lips; etc.

The Timing and Nature of a Reaction

A serious allergic reaction may often occur very soon after a medication is taken, in most cases within the first hour. (Onset at times may not begin until after one hour, if the medication is taken orally, or with food.) It's seen even with medications that you have previously tolerated well, without difficulty. The reaction can worsen if the offending drug is continued.

The other type of reaction, which is much more common, is delayed. It's often less severe—but not always. An allergy to a drug can emerge up to approximately seventy-two hours later. The delayed reaction usually manifests as a rash that appears a day or two (or longer) after ingesting the drug, and which often spreads across the skin. The rash may be itchy. Delayed hypersensitivity reaction, a particular type of delayed reaction, often unfolds over days and even weeks: It happens when the T cell, which is part of the immune system, finally identifies the invader (the drug you've taken), triggering a release of chemicals. The skin is usually affected and a rash develops, one that is either flat and reddened or elevated and bumpy. This reaction may also include blistering and peeling. This condition commonly brings about fever, and may also affect kidneys, lungs, liver, and heart. Some of the drugs most likely to trigger delayed hypersensitivity reaction: antibiotics (e.g., penicillin; sulfa drugs in prescription topical cream, for burns), antiseizure medications (e.g., Lamictal), and medication for depression and gout.

Often, a higher dose of a drug can increase the risk of a delayed reaction.

ONSET OF A DRUG REACTION

Acute: within the first hour of taking the drug
Accelerated: between one and twenty-four hours after taking the drug
Delayed: more than twenty-four hours after taking the drug

Drug reaction is the reason behind 5 percent of all hospital admissions. In-hospital drug reactions happen in 10 to 20 percent of patients, and 20 percent of those are severe.

Serious drug reactions can happen with OTC medication, too—for example, oral decongestants combined with antihistamines, taken for rapid relief of nasal congestion, may cause a variety of new problems, such as rapid heart rate, increased sweating, increased blood pressure (which can be associated with a small rise in stroke risk), and increased urinary retention in patients with enlarged prostate; it may worsen certain types of glaucoma. Other side effects include insomnia, nervousness, and tremors. Because decongestant may trigger adverse effects, I emphasize to many of my patients that the letter "D" in decongestant also stands, potentially, for "Do not take"—at least for some.

Allergy of all kinds, including drug allergy, may result in anaphylaxis, a potentially life-threatening reaction that may affect two or more organ systems at once (evidenced, for instance, when you experience both breathing difficulty *and* rash). The likeliest drugs to trigger anaphylaxis are antibiotics. There are increasing reports that chemotherapy drugs and monoclonal antibodies (a form of targeted immunotherapy, used in place of traditional chemotherapy) may cause it, too: While anaphylaxis is likeliest to occur (if it occurs at all, which is not typical) when the patient is receiving chemotherapy, at times it can take up to several hours.

The Skin: An Early-Warning System

The most common symptom of drug allergy is rash—often called (simply enough) "drug rash," with the skin turning red and irritated (hives). Other skin-related symptoms include generalized itchiness; swelling (of the face, tongue, throat, hands, feet); sweating and/or flushing. As the reaction progresses, throat tightness, trouble swallowing, wheezing, trouble breathing, cramps, abdominal pain, vomiting, diarrhea, dizziness, feeling faint, and a drop in blood pressure may occur.

In rare circumstances, a severe skin rash develops into a blister and the skin peels, a potentially life-threatening condition that must be treated like a severe burn.

Here's the range of drug-induced skin reactions I see in my office:

- Generalized rash, which can appear as flat or raised (bumpy), often on both sides of the body in matching distribution (e.g., both forearms). The most common drugs responsible include beta-lactam antibiotics, such as penicillin, sulfa antibiotics or sulfonamides, and anticonvulsants.
- Localized or fixed-location rash; typically appears on the face and/or genital region; interestingly, these reactions recur in the same location upon repeated ingestion of the drug. Itchiness is less common with this reaction. Commonly implicated drugs are penicillin, tetracycline, and sulfonamides. Unfortunately, after subsiding, this type of rash can leave the skin darker in color.
- Hives and angioedema (swelling of the skin), featuring varying sizes of hives. This is one of the more common medication reactions. Drug culprits typically include antibiotics, especially penicillin, intravenous X-ray contrast agents used in CT scans and MRIs, and anesthetics. The reaction generally lasts less than one day, and resolves promptly when the drug is stopped.
- Redness, swelling, scaliness, pigment changes (darker or lighter) where itchiness is present; this type of reaction may be triggered

by local anesthetic agents (e.g., injectable lidocaine or Novocain used at the dental office), as well as topical creams and ointments that contain neomycin, typically used to prevent a skin infection. Patch testing can be used as a diagnostic tool to identify the sensitizing agent.

- Blisters that may even resemble a burn affecting up to one-third of the skin surface; loss of superficial layer of skin; also associated with lesions in the mouth; this is potentially a life-threatening reaction known as Stevens-Johnson syndrome, or, if a more extensive area of skin is affected, toxic epidermal necrolysis. Both are rare conditions that require immediate medical attention.

Getting It vs. Not Getting It

Why do some people get drug allergy and others don't? While the answer is not clear, some factors appear to increase risk: genetics; body chemistry; previous allergies such as hay fever and sometimes asthma; frequent/copious if intermittent drug exposure (e.g., you already took a course of drug therapy); age; and whether the drug was taken via injection or intravenously rather than in pill form. A large study in the journal *Allergy* reported that women may be more likely than men to have a drug allergy, especially to antibiotics.

The key is to minimize unnecessary medications when possible and to work diligently to try to prevent reactions before they occur.

Other possible risk factors for drug allergy include the presence of certain diseases, including viral infections such as Epstein-Barr or HIV. It's unclear, however, if the heightened risk is due to an immunological abnormality or because the individual has been bombarded with numerous medicines.

You may not react to a drug the very first time you are exposed. However, you may have taken a similar drug in the past, or maybe you actually took the drug before and didn't know that you did. The next time you are exposed to the same drug, you can develop allergic symp-

> ## Keep a Record
>
> ■
>
> Inform your doctor of any adverse reaction you've had while taking medication, currently or in the past. Keep handy a list of drugs you're on, noting unusual reactions. Are you someone who ought to wear a special bracelet alerting others to your serious medication allergy?

toms to the medication. Being exposed to a similar chemical in a cosmetic or the like could be sufficient to sensitize you.

If the number one strategy for dealing with allergy today is avoidance—and it is—then it helps a potentially drug-allergic individual to know how best to reduce the likelihood of expressing, or developing, medication allergies and reactions.

1. If you have a reaction to a drug, it is important to understand its class or type of medication (e.g., a statin, a commonly prescribed cholesterol-lowering agent, a class of migraine medication), or drugs otherwise similar to that one, because you may well want to steer clear of them, too. Such related drugs, along with the original culprit, should be avoided unless a "drug challenge" deems it safe. (This procedure should be done only when appropriate, and in the presence of an experienced allergist trained in the procedure.) This situation is often true with penicillin and similar class antibiotics in the extended penicillin family.

2. If you react to aspirin or one of the many non-steroidal anti-inflammatory (NSAID) agents, then it's essential to consult a practitioner (such as an allergist) for advice on whether it's appropriate or safe to take another type of NSAID for pain and anti-inflammatory relief. In most cases, it is safe to use an alternative drug (e.g., low-dose acetaminophen).

3. If you are allergic to a medication, your options include working

with your health care provider to identify a suitable alternative; consulting with an allergist and possibly undergoing a drug challenge test; or in extreme cases, undergoing one of several medication desensitization protocols, performed at a facility with staff expert at these procedures.

Drugs We're Commonly Allergic To

ANTIBIOTICS—PENICILLIN

The number one cause of drug allergy, penicillin, may affect as many as one in ten people. Serious reactions are common. And I have found what other allergists have found: Many people who believe they have a penicillin allergy, don't. (This is confirmed through testing.)

Symptoms of penicillin allergy may vary in their presentation but can include rash and hives, swelling (usually around the face) and tightness in the throat, wheezing, coughing, and breathing trouble. Through skin testing and, if available, one's previous medical history with penicillin, an allergist can help to determine if taking penicillin is safe.

There are antibiotics similar to penicillin, such as cephalosporin, which are commonly prescribed; yet these, too, may cause a reaction in someone with a penicillin allergy, especially if they've had a reaction more recently (within the previous ten years). If a cephalosporin antibiotic is needed for treatment, an allergist can help to determine if skin testing, drug challenge or desensitization may be appropriate.

Young children may develop mild rash or hives in response to antibiotics, especially amoxicillin; when the child is also suffering from viral infection, this reaction will happen even more frequently. Note that developing such a rash does not indicate with certainty that she's allergic to amoxicillin and similar antibiotics. Consult with your pediatrician and/or an allergist for proper advice and/or treatment.

Most people "outgrow" penicillin allergy. A reaction once does not guarantee a reaction the next time, especially after a prolonged period has lapsed. But the decision to try penicillin, if you have a history of reaction to it, should never be made without the advice of an experienced allergist, and often only after a negative drug challenge.

Some risk factors that *may* indicate an allergy to penicillin and other antibiotics:

1. age
2. multiple courses of penicillin antibiotics
3. history of having allergic reactions to other medications
4. history of other allergic conditions

ANTIBIOTICS—SULFA

Up to 3 percent of the population has an allergy to sulfa drugs (also called sulfonamides). Antibiotics that contain sulfa drugs include Septra and Bactrim (sulfamethoxazole-trimethoprim) and Pediazole (erythromycin-sulfisoxazole). They may trigger an allergic reaction. Some non-antibiotic medications, such as some diuretics, including furosemide, contain a chemical resemblance to sulfa drugs, but are often well tolerated by sulfa antibiotic-allergic patients. If you have a sulfa allergy, consult with an allergist about using other medications since they may pose a risk.

An allergy to sulfa drugs is not typically an issue for those who can't

Did You Know?

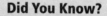

Sulfa drugs were the first antibiotics to enjoy widespread use in the United States, starting in the 1930s. For many years before penicillin, they were the only effective and available—though at times dangerously unregulated—antibiotic.

A Not Uncommon Reaction

∎

Up to one-third of people who take an ACE inhibitor, a commonly prescribed blood pressure/cardiac medication, get a persistent cough. Others may suffer a more serious reaction: angioedema, a sudden swelling of the mouth, tongue, and lips and, in more severe cases, closing of the throat. This condition is more common in women and African-Americans. ACE inhibitor–related angioedema may occur shortly after starting the drug but in some cases the reaction can be delayed, even occurring only after months or years!

---

tolerate sulfites, which are used as preservatives in various foods (especially frozen) and are also found in wine.

NSAIDS, SUCH AS ASPIRIN, IBUPROFEN, OR NAPROXEN

Sensitivity to aspirin or other NSAIDs is not uncommon in asthmatic adults and in those with (benign) nasal polyps. Symptoms include stuffy nose, wheezing, and breathing difficulty. Other reactions to these analgesics may include hives and/or angioedema. Patients with asthma who are unable to tolerate aspirin may also have difficulty in taking other anti-inflammatory agents such as ibuprofen and naproxen. Some may be able to tolerate celecoxib (Celebrex) and acetaminophen (Tylenol, in low dose) as anti-inflammatory medications; however, seek the advice of an experienced drug allergy expert.

Other trigger drugs include quinolone antibiotics, chemotherapy medications, neurologic blocking drugs used during anesthesia, anticonvulsants, blood products, opiates, and topical steroid creams and ointments. Allergic reaction can also happen to biological agents, which are often used in the treatment of various autoimmune conditions.

> ## Antibiotics May Not Be the Answer
>
> ■
>
> Viruses, not bacteria, are the cause of many sinus infections, thus antibiotics cannot treat them successfully.

Photosensitivity

Photosensitivity, or photodermatitis, refers to skin that is inflamed by sunlight, facilitated by the interaction of a drug. It affects only a small number of people. In some, it resembles sunburn.

There are two types of drug-induced photosensitivity. In the first, "phototoxic," the drug is activated by exposure to UV light, causing rash chiefly at the site of the light exposure. It generally resolves promptly once the offending drug is discontinued. Some common phototoxic drugs:

- antibiotics (quinolones, tetracycline, sulfa drugs)
- malaria medicines
- chemotherapeutic agents
- heart medicines (diuretics)
- diabetes medicines (sulfonylureas, glyburide)
- analgesic or pain medicines (NSAIDs)
- acne medicines (isotretinoins)
- psychiatric treatments (tricyclic antidepressants, phenothiazine)

The second type of photosensitivity, "photoallergic," is also brought about by the combination of drug and UV light exposure which, after several days, causes a change in the drug's chemical structure; the immune system reacts as if it's being attacked, causing an allergic response. This form of photosensitivity may resemble eczema and often persists. It is also more commonly associated with topical medications—that is, drugs applied to the skin. Common photosensitizing medications (not a complete list):

- antibiotics
- diuretics
- retinoids (for various dermatological conditions, including acne)
- hypoglycemics (lowers glucose levels in the blood)
- neuroleptics (anticonvulsants)
- cardiovascular agents
- fragrances (musk, 6-methylcoumarin)

Various foods may also be triggers for photosensitivity. When certain fruits, vegetables, and other foods, such as celery, lime, mango peel, and parsley, among others, are exposed to the skin, they can cause a phototoxic reaction.

Adverse Drug Reactions That Are Not Allergy

Many people who believe they have drug allergy don't. As noted earlier, one study found that the vast majority of patients who thought they were allergic to penicillin were not. Another study showed that allergy to local anesthetics during dental and/or other procedures was "more myth than reality"; that "most adverse reactions to local anesthetics are due to non-allergic factors . . . [and] true immune-based 'allergic' type or IgE-mediated reactions are exceedingly rare."

However, there are genuine and unpleasant drug reactions (and worse) of the *non*-allergic type, and these are actually considerably more common than the allergic.

The most obvious case? The side effects of a drug that are to be expected, and are listed on the packaging. For example, drowsiness is a side effect felt by many people who take antihistamines: That's not an allergic reaction. When amoxicillin is taken during infectious mononucleosis, rash will develop in a significant number of patients. Chemo-

> ## Touchy
>
> ■
>
> With some individuals, applying a medication topically (cream, ointment) produces allergic-type contact dermatitis, a rash caused by a specific chemical that reacts with the skin.

therapy drugs often lead to nausea, vomiting, and hair loss. The intravenous contrast agents (formerly known as dyes) used for enhancing the quality and interpretation of various CT or MRI scans can lead to itching, flushing, red skin, and other symptoms, including drop in blood pressure (though that's rare); though these symptoms are similar to anaphylaxis, they are due to a different mechanism.

There can also be side effects that happen precisely because of a drug interaction—that is, the patient is taking more than one drug, and experiencing something from the unique commingling of the medications.

Here's another example of an adverse non-allergic drug reaction—something we'd call an "indirect effect" rather than an "expected effect": Antibiotics can kill normal bacteria in the bowel, leading to intestinal irritation, stomach cramps, and diarrhea. This, too, is not the result of allergy.

Aside from these possibilities, there is also "drug intolerance," which is not an allergic condition. An example? If you take opioid medications (narcotic painkillers) like morphine, you may feel nausea.

Diagnosis

Drug allergies, as you can see, are often tough to identify. The symptoms of a drug reaction—such as rashes, hives, and wheezing—may look like that of other diseases. What's more, people often take multiple medications so it may not be apparent that one of them is being rejected (or, after years free of problem, has suddenly become rejected). The one drug allergy that we can reliably diagnose: penicillin, and drugs like it—a good thing, since penicillin is the single biggest cause of drug allergy. A skin test administered by an allergist can resolve the question. For non-penicillin-type antibiotics, skin testing is also helpful but needs to be confirmed with an oral drug challenge.

To figure out the source of other potential drug allergies, it's up to my patient and me to leverage her information to get at why she's having a reaction. The story and circumstances behind a reaction need to be as complete as possible. The solution is in the details, and the sequence of events is important. We're trying to find pieces to a puzzle.

Some questions I would ask her:

- Is this the first time a reaction has occurred, or is there a prior pattern of reaction?
- Do you suspect a drug you're taking is the cause of your reaction?
- If so, how long have you been taking it?
- Are you still taking it?
- Did you experience symptoms soon after you first took the drug?
- How long was the duration between first taking the drug and the reaction?
- What were the symptoms and how long before they went away?
- Did the reaction resolve completely?
- Do you take other prescription medications or OTC meds?
- How about herbal medications, vitamins, or mineral supplements?
- Do you have any other current illnesses, conditions, or infections?
- Was the skin involved in the reaction (rash, itch, hives, swelling, and/or flushing)?
- Were there abdominal or gastrointestinal symptoms (nausea, abdominal discomfort, bloating, excess gas, vomiting, diarrhea) and, if so, when did they begin after starting on the medication?

- Did you experience any trouble swallowing, choking, throat tightness, chest pain, breathing, wheezing, or coughing?
- How did you relieve your discomfort?
- Have you ever reacted to another drug?
- Do you have any history of atopic dermatitis (eczema)?

Depending on the answers, I may ask my patient to bring in one or more of the medications she's taking. I may recommend a full drug allergy evaluation, including skin testing, to help pinpoint the risk of developing a severe, perhaps delayed reaction, which can involve multiple organ systems.

If I think you have a drug allergy, it's often unnecessary and unwise to do further testing. When I think you're not allergic to a particular drug, I may elect to do a drug challenge to confirm that. You're given a small amount of the drug in question, in gradual doses. This evaluation may take place in the office or a hospital setting, and should be performed only when the circumstances warrant its use, and all potential safety parameters are considered, because it comes with inherent risk.

As it is with all suspected allergy triggers, if you have a drug allergy or suspect one, cease taking the drug. You may also want to avoid drugs very similar to the one in question. Make sure that you tell your doctor of any possible drug allergy and the symptoms you experienced. If anaphylaxis is a concern, consider wearing a medical alert bracelet identifying your allergy, or at least carrying on you a filled-out, wallet-size

Picture This

■

Photograph your adverse skin reaction. It may fade or disappear before your appointment with the allergist, and if he or she can't get a good look at the problem on your body, it helps at least to have some visual record.

Secondary Problems

■

Every time Shannon had a headache, it seemed to be accompanied by swollen lips. At the pharmacy she asked for some fast-acting antihistamine for the swelling. The pharmacist asked her what she was taking before the lips swelled up. "Nothing," she said. "Just a plain ibuprofen liquid gel capsule for the headache."

And that was it: Analgesic or pain pills like it, among the most common medication around, are a leading cause of swelling of the face and/or lips. This is not well-known among patients.

What to do instead for your headache? Low-dose acetaminophen can be a good alternative for mild aches, pain and/or fever.

---

anaphylaxis card listing your drug allergies. Your doctor can prescribe an epinephrine auto-injector.

Drug Desensitization

For those with allergies to multiple antibiotics, what do you do? One study recommends that you take antibiotics only for infections that are proven (via culture or X-ray); if you have sinusitis, bronchitis, or otitis,

---

Don't Spend Your Money on That Ointment!

■

I do not recommend using OTC skin products with diphenhydramine (an antihistamine). That antihistamine can be extremely effective when taken in oral form or as an injection. As a topical cream? Its effectiveness remains largely unproven.

Contrast Reactions (Injectable X-Ray Imaging Agents)

■

If you are a woman, have a history of allergy or asthma, or previously experienced a reaction to an injectable contrast agent, then you have an increased risk of a radiocontrast reaction. You can lessen the risk by taking a recommended medication (e.g., antihistamines, steroids) before exposure to a contrast agent. Consult with an experienced medical professional or allergist before receiving a contrast agent, especially if you are at risk.

---

forgo antibiotics altogether since they are typically not helpful for those conditions.

But if you do need an antibiotic, there is very likely one out there to which you are *not* allergic. There are choices.

Another possibility, drug desensitization, has now been standardized for many medications including chemotherapy, monoclonal antibodies, and antibiotics. Desensitization is really meant only for those who need to take a particular drug where no similarly effective therapy exists. The offending drug is given to you in increasing amounts until you tolerate the needed dose with minimal side effects. The desensitizing process is often performed in a hospital, where help is immediately available if a problem arises. The record of safety and effectiveness of drug desensitization is excellent. This therapy has saved the lives of countless patients who needed a particular medication as a first-line therapy.

If desensitization works and you make it through the cycle—say, a round of chemotherapy—it does not necessarily mean that you have successfully desensitized to that drug forever. Should you need a second cycle of chemo, you'll need to go through the desensitization process again.

Desensitization is also a possibility for patients allergic to aspirin, and for whom the medication would be beneficial for their asthma, sinus disease/nasal polyposis, or cardiac disease.

I won't go into further detail here on the specifics of drug desensitization because it's beyond the scope of this chapter and book, but it's important to mention that it can be an option for some people, in some situations. When any adverse drug reaction happens, both allergist and patient are after the same goals: to confirm the diagnosis, come up with a good plan for managing the reaction, and prevent future occurrences—while also figuring out which alternative medication will do the job that was needed in the first place.

New Ways

Chapter 10

Managing Allergy and Asthma, Today and Tomorrow

Terry, an ob-gyn, came to my office, having suffered from hives for months. I talked with her, made some observations about her condition, took some history. Before embarking on any diagnostic tests, though, I noted that she had undergone not one but two recent stressful life events—a mediocre review at work, her boyfriend expressing doubts about their relationship—at almost exactly the same time that her hives first appeared. I recommended that she work with Bonnie, a colleague and a talented psychiatrist well-versed in various mind-body approaches, from mindfulness training to dance therapy to yoga to cognitive behavioral therapy.

Terry agreed. Bonnie presented her with a range of self-help possibilities. Terry particularly took to a mix of daily aerobics and once-weekly yoga, along with her prescribed antihistamines. Within a couple of weeks, the severity and frequency of Terry's hives were dramatically improved; within six weeks, they were gone.

I realize that this sort of non-medication intervention does not work in every case, or in most. And when it *does* work, it won't always be this easy, quick, or complete. Still, I hope that this illustrates how some disease conditions, which often manifest on the skin, may have a psychological component; and how our understanding of and approach to these conditions are evolving, thanks in part to the emerging science of neuroimmunology, which incorporates numerous mind-body concepts.

It's not hard to see how emotional state affects the skin: Think of when we blush, and what must go on underneath the skin to cause that change. Or the inverse: Think of how skin-to-skin contact enjoyed by a newborn and her mother immediately after birth obviously affects mood and occasions a release of chemicals.

Physiology and psychology intersect all the time. Stress can impact the immune system. For people like Terry, a correlation appears to exist between periods of persistent, heightened stress and flare-ups of a skin condition.

Mood can also affect us positively. Patients who expressed comparatively modest feelings of stress in the month leading up to their surgical procedure registered higher levels of IL-1, a chemical of the immune system that is involved in the "stress response."

The relatively new field of psychodermatology explores this "cross talk" happening with various skin immune responses—the neuroimmunologic communication of receptors and chemical messengers, and how their actions can interfere with, or enhance, the skin's normal functioning. Those in the field are hoping to use their findings to identify newer therapies to complement and/or improve existing ones (e.g., anti-allergic and anti-inflammatory drugs, topical medications). I'm hopeful that complementary or alternative strategies like these—and there are many—broaden our toolkit. We're constantly on the watch for ways to improve and speed up relief, both the physiological variety and the psychological/emotional one. Hives, eczema, and the like may wear us out; we want to feel as if we have some agency in our healing; we don't want to feel as if it's only about finding the right meds. The skin works in tandem with our "central stress" response system, which oversees a broad array of tightly regulated hormones and substances ready to be released, triggering a cycle of actions responsible for numerous inflammatory skin diseases. Psychodermatology appreciates the mind-body connection, and that there's a range of steps we might take to help improve or reduce symptoms related to allergy. Researchers are looking to see how, or if, neuroimmunological mechanisms may be at least partly responsible for outbreaks. They are exploring how stress can lead to overstimulation of the nerves in the skin, leading to the release of neuro-peptides (chemical messengers that bind to receptors in the brain and the entire nervous system), which can lead to the activation of mast cells, then the release of histamine, and the itchiness that characterizes so many skin conditions. It is my sincere hope that we will finally come to understand enough to better serve those, in particular, whose chronic hives have no identifiable cause, and who suffer from it for years and years. Researchers are looking at how psychosocial and emotional triggers can affect complex neurologic and hormonal pathways, worsening or triggering skin conditions such as hives, flushing of skin, eczema, and more.

In medical school, young doctors learn in embryology that the brain and skin are connected very early on in development: Both skin and nerves come from the same layer of the embryo. Our skin is alive; our nerves allow us to feel things touching our skin. *Our own development suggests a brain-skin connection.* There are brain-body connections. We need to understand them better.

In my practice, I have seen this play out many times. Terry's case is hardly isolated. Peter, an MBA candidate at a New York–area university, suffered greatly from persistent eczema, which worsened the further he got in the semester. Working with a psychologist, along with his continued dermatology management, which included moisturizers, prescription emollients, and topical steroid creams to reduce eczema, helped Peter to return to some normalcy.

School stress also got to Anna, a premed college junior: Upcoming midterms turned her asthma from something controllable to a condition debilitating enough to make her suspend her daily exercise routine. Working with a therapist on anxiety-reducing behaviors helped manage her distress, until she achieved near-perfect control of her respiratory symptoms within weeks.

Years ago, I authored two papers on the effect of anxiety on asthma.

Will That Be on the Final?

■

It's no stretch to include "allergic disease" in the same sentence with "chronic stress." Several years ago, some clever researchers, studying a population of college students, measured their count of eosinophils (a type of white blood cell associated with some allergic conditions) before and after allergen exposure to the cells, at different points in the semester, including midway and again during finals. The eosinophil count was higher, and its elevation longer-lasting, during final exams. It was just a single study but it reveals what many of us see in our practices: The worsening, or onset, of allergic symptoms is very often associated with chronic stress and/or anxiety.

In my practice, I sometimes use a self-reporting, surprisingly helpful "anxiety scoring system." As an allergy detective, if I gather information about my patients to deduce the cause of their frequently elusive condition, why wouldn't I include their thoughts and emotions, which are powerful and consuming enough to affect sleep patterns, appetite, clarity, capacity to fight back—indeed, the very chemicals that we release? If so many of the conditions I deal with now are multifactorial, isn't it likely that the mind, the major functional unit of the central nervous system, is occasionally one of those factors?

Studies have shown that the skin's permeability barrier, designed to keep out harmful substances and prevent fluid loss from layers of skin cells (eczema happens when this function fails), can be disrupted by chronic negative stress.

Numerous mind-body and "alternative" strategies have been studied. For example, biofeedback has been used in medical settings when behavior modification is called for; I've worked closely with practitioners expert in this technique who have helped asthma patients control their condition over time.

In this chapter, I am here to highlight nonconventional, alternative ways to deal with allergy and asthma, approaches that complement your medication and medical management. With patients, I look for the strategy that targets their particular situation. We'll explore the non-medication strategies that not only provide relief of discomfort but also may improve their overall health.

Many of the best researchers in allergy and health believe as much as I do: There are proactive, preventive paths for managing and reducing a host of allergic conditions. But do we have support for this belief that's more than anecdotal? In many cases, it's only fair to middling—as yet. Where studies *do* provide support, the reported benefits are—so far, anyway—not transformative but rather more modest. And the benefits don't help every individual, every time, across all allergic and asthmatic conditions.

I readily admit that there is very limited evidence that certain integrative or complementary and alternative medical (CAM) approaches—traditional Chinese medicine, Ayurvedic medicine, acupuncture, manual therapy massage, to name a few—aid in allergy and/or asthma management. It must be said, however, that some of my patients believe they have derived benefit; and the much larger anecdotal pool of individuals being helped by these techniques (e.g., improvements ranging from less itchiness and reduced reliance on medication to reduced anxiety) cannot be denied. Traditional Chinese medicine (TCM), after all, has been a therapeutic staple for centuries in East Asia to treat asthma.

Although many nontraditional approaches have been around for a long time, there is clearly a need for more and better controlled studies, with larger sample sizes, to prove their efficacy. To take one example, the risks and benefits of TCM, though partly non-medicinal, should be considered carefully. With herbal remedies comes a risk of nonstandard or incorrect plant selection, preparation and dosing, as well as the possibility of adulteration (e.g., with ephedra, heavy metals like lead). Consumer warnings have been issued by the FDA to not rely on homeopathic products marketed for asthma relief. The FDA has not evaluated these products, regardless of their claims that they are "safe and even effective." There are proven, effective treatments for allergies, eczema, and asthma that have been rigorously studied, regulated by the FDA, and withstood the test of time. While you may desire a more alternative approach, these proven therapies should be viewed as first-line treatment options.

I am by nature a cautious man and practitioner. But I am comfortable introducing you to many of the most current, exciting possibilities around allergy and asthma care. Just because not enough study has been done to provide ironclad, 100 percent proof, a possible breakthrough approach should not be shelved when it potentially provides great benefit, while also ensuring adequate safety. However, the risks and benefits of selecting such an agent over an established product or technique that has met such a standard need to be carefully considered; there may be harm in selecting something unproven that better aligns with your personal health beliefs. As health-care providers, we walk a cautious line to "do no harm"; we also want to find a hopeful, shared vision. Therefore, even if some mind-body practice or dietary change does not result in noticeable alleviation of allergy or asthma symptoms, so long as no harm is done (directly, or indirectly through a "wrong" choice that worsens the condition), my patient may get some overall health benefit. My own interpretation of a contemporary, pro-integrative medicine focus is, by definition, not limited to drugs and medical procedures as the ultimate, sole answer.

Let's start with the subject about which I get the most questions: diet.

Diet

What do we know so far about how—or whether—dietary changes (more fresh fruits, vegetables, fish, etc.) that we're told are beneficial for overall health truly reduce allergy or asthma symptoms, or the progression of the disease? Not as much as we'd like—or, rather, studies on the consumption of antioxidants; vitamins A, C, D, and E; soy isoflavones;

and more have not yet proved a meaningful positive effect on adults or children. (These studies certainly have not shown any negative effect; and they have previously and widely been shown to improve health overall.) Despite provocative headlines and research claims, what remains unknown is the exact amount of vitamins and other dietary factors that may be beneficial.

Measurements of low vitamin D levels appear to be associated with worsening asthma, and some limited data from Australia suggest that low vitamin D levels may be associated with development of food allergy. But until recently, we couldn't yet say, with scientific backing, that the converse was also true—that by taking more vitamin D, you'll potentially decrease the severity of your asthma or allergy. After all, it could be that levels of vitamin D are not precisely synched with asthma or select allergic conditions, and there's some threshold of vitamin D concentration only below which allergy or asthma is affected; it could be that other factors play a role for the impact of vitamin D level to matter. (Your vitamin D level can be identified with a simple blood test.)

A recent survey of studies, however, concluded that greater vitamin D in utero *does* correlate with lowered risk of childhood asthma, "wheeze," and respiratory tract infection. It points to further evidence of the potential effectiveness of nutritional intervention. What we hoped might be the case . . . appears to be the case!

That's what we want to find out: If any of these vitamins or other nutrients have, in a word, a prophylactic or preventive effect (or a harmful effect or no effect) on changing the course of one's allergies and asthma. If that turns out to be provably true, then it would be a tremendous development. We're still working off of sometimes inconclusive, generally modest claims such as "High plasma carotenoid[1] concentrations [in] a diet high in various fruits and vegetables *might* have a protective effect on allergic rhinitis in adulthood."[2]

---

1. Carotenoids include carrots, dark green leafy vegetables, sweet potato, tomato, squash, melon, peppers, and broccoli.
2. The difficulty is in understanding how to design the perfect study to prove conclusively that something "works." At times, it's more than difficult—it's impossible. We're

I'm glad to say that, despite my own professional reticence and that of the scientific and medical community to say something like, "Eat this super-healthy diet and your eczema or allergy and asthma symptoms will disappear!" we are accumulating evidence for the possible benefits of eating certain foods. We must keep in mind the difference between claims of prevention and treatment. For example, when we observe the association between vitamin D and allergic disease, is the first data point—taking in more vitamin D, or having a generally higher vitamin D level—precursor to the second data point—lower occurrence of allergy? If so, vitamin D would appear to have a potential preventive effect, and we might advocate for a change in dietary habit *before* the onset of the disease (primary prevention). On the other hand, a study might show an association between vitamin D level and the improvement of a known allergic condition (secondary or tertiary prevention).

Here's a roundup of some possibly allergy/asthma-healthy substances.

CAN DIET AND VITAMINS IMPACT ALLERGY AND ASTHMA IN CHILDREN AND ADULTS?

- A German study among adults showed that a high content of n-3 fatty acids in the diet was associated with a lowered risk of allergic sensitization and allergic rhinitis. Foods rich in those fatty acids include flaxseed and flaxseed oil, salmon and other fish (particularly fatty types), chia seed, walnut and walnut oil, soybean and soybean oil, spinach, pumpkin seed, rapeseed (canola) oil, and olive oil. A diet rich in omega-fatty acids, which are abundant in the Mediterranean diet, also provides benefit to asthmatics, particularly those with exercise-induced asthma. The Mediterranean diet has been associated in studies with other

---

frequently left with studies that cannot show cause and effect, but only "association" or "correlation" in a particular direction. This is one of the frustrating complexities of modern medicine: Often, there are limitations to the quality of the available evidence. It is this evidence we use, often cautiously, to best advise our patients.

health benefits such as lower cardiovascular risk, but that's different from proven cause and effect.

- Vitamin E, found in many edible nuts, may have a possible antioxidant effect on inflammation in the airways of the lungs, fighting infection, and/or hastening recovery after exercise.
- One clinical trial identified a possible association between supplementing with the mineral magnesium and improvement in asthma control and patient-reported quality of life.
- Other studies point to the possible constructive impact that antioxidants and the mineral zinc could have on young children with asthma and/or wheezing.

While these may yield minor benefits (if that), there's reason to believe more, and more profound, linkage between healthy diet and fewer/milder symptoms are in our future. Remember, the quality of these studies and other research is variable. A study published in *Cell Reports* showed a link in mice between gut bacteria and the development of food allergies. Rodents who from birth were fed a diet that was average in sugar, fiber content, and calories had more severe peanut allergies than mice whose diet was high in fiber.

Is there such a thing as an anti-asthma diet? If inflammation of lung tissue (among other areas) is a defining aspect of asthma, then would an anti-inflammatory diet provide symptom relief and reduce the risk of future attacks? There is no clinically proven diet recommended for helping to manage asthma but some other select studies feature potentially beneficial nutritional strategies. Again, a caution: The following is "not yet ready for prime time"—but nonetheless worth noting:

Coffee. Caffeine is chemically similar to theophylline (from the same plant family as cocoa), a bronchodilator previously used in asthma treatment. One analysis reported that "even small amounts of caffeine can improve lung function for up to four hours." Can this improvement be felt with a "practical" amount of caffeine? I advise caution: The volume of coffee (milligrams of caffeine) needed for bronchodilation improvement would likely result in major side effects. Before I recommend that my patients add another daily trip to their local Starbucks, more studies are needed to confirm safety and effectiveness. (News cycles are full of stories that fail to detail actual benefit, who might benefit, or what dosage/quantity was tested before an effect was observed. These are important distinctions.) Keep in mind not to overdo your coffee intake or you may need treatment for another condition—acid reflux!

Oranges. Asthmatic children who ate vitamin C–rich fruits, such as oranges, wheezed less, according to a preliminary study.

Apples. Phytochemicals and flavonoids (like catechins, quercetin, etc.) have been studied for their ability to improve lung capacity. A study from London's St. George's Hospital, published in *Thorax*, reported that "eating an apple a day may be good for the lungs, and reported in those eating five or more apples a week had slightly better lung function." (However, it was also speculated that these individuals may be more likely to eat apples to begin with.)

Fish and fish oils have been shown in some studies to possibly reduce inflammation. A Finnish study found that early introduction of

Go Green

■

A study found that for those suffering from allergic rhinitis (specifically, allergy to Japanese cedar pollen), if they began consuming Benifuuki, a type of green tea, a month and a half before pollen season, their symptoms were reduced. What was the magic substance? It's thought that it might be the catechins in the green tea leaf.

Can we take this as a good sign? Yes—but also, for now, a limited one. There is no evidence yet that the medicinal powers of Benifuuki are true for all varieties of green tea leaf, or that those allergic to other seasonal pollens would benefit. We'll wait to find that out—and hope for similar or even better results.

fish into the diet was associated with a small decrease in the risk of multiple allergies by age five.

The findings of several studies have led to the conclusion that important aspects of the Mediterranean diet could benefit those who follow it; since those who adhere to it have shown a relative lack of allergic symptoms, researchers speculate that the diet may provide some protective effect against the development of atopy and asthma in kids.

ALLERGY/ASTHMA, DIET . . . AND WEIGHT?

We know that people with greater body mass index (BMI) or risk for obesity appear to be at greater risk for asthma, and have more severe symptoms. What happens to their asthma when they lose weight?

A review of four studies looked at this question. The authors found that weight loss strategies in overweight and/or obese patients with asthma *did* improve control of their asthma. The diets were associated with fewer symptoms, including less need for rescue inhalers. In my practice, I have observed firsthand how emphasis on a prudent diet combined with exercise appeared to help many patients to control their weight—not to mention accruing all the other potential health and life benefits one gets from eating better.

At least, that's been my observation.

Nutrition experts at England's University of Nottingham studied the diets of more than 300,000 children and adolescents, plus the parents of more than 180,000 school-aged children. In the journal *Thorax*, the authors reported that teens who consumed fast food more than three times per week had a 33 percent increase in risk of developing eczema, hay fever, or severe asthma. Children and adolescents who ate three or more servings of fruit per week reduced their likelihood of developing allergies and/or eczema by 10 to 14 percent.

The researchers' explanation for their findings? It could be that fast food promotes inflammation, which in turn is associated with the development of eczema and asthma. (Asthma is the most common chronic inflammatory childhood disease.) Does that mean that a diet rich in fresh fruit, vegetables, fish, and other foods that do not promote inflammation helps someone with eczema or asthma to tame symptoms? Does it help someone without those conditions to avoid them?

Again: The science does not yet support the thesis that good/ improved diet = less allergy and asthma. But my years of practice tell me it often has a positive effect (and never a negative one). The benefit will vary person to person, and there are other factors that influence the outcomes. However, I think that the answer here is unequivocally yes. Your diet makes a difference. Eating healthy foods makes you generally healthier—more energetic, perhaps putting you in a better mood, which better arms you to deal with whatever comes along, including symptoms and setbacks, including heightened stress and other challenging conditions characteristic of asthma and various allergic conditions.

PROBIOTICS

Do probiotics—live, beneficial bacteria and yeast, the "good" kind of bacteria—benefit our gastrointestinal system? They are thought to promote wellness by replacing some bad bacteria with good ones, and restoring balance between the two types. Probiotics exist as supplements and are also abundant in various foods: certain fruits and juices; fermented foods; some dairy. If they can keep your gut healthy, could that lead to a reduction in allergy, eczema, and perhaps asthma symptoms? Might they even stop progression of the disease?

One or two studies provide hopeful results; another one or two or more show no meaningful allergy reduction in high-risk children when their mothers took probiotic supplements. Yet another study found no benefit in the treatment of eczema.

The prevailing belief in the research community? There's simply not enough evidence-based data to support recommending that expectant mothers take probiotics (or prebiotics) for preventing allergic disease in newborns, or that young children will benefit. There's not enough data pointing to the benefit of probiotics in the treatment of any allergic condition.

The one thing we can say for sure on this subject: We need more large, properly designed studies to resolve this important question. Few of the studies evaluating probiotic use in the prevention or treatment of allergic conditions have used the same type of probiotic, or dosage, making it challenging to recommend which type of probiotic a patient might use, how much, and for how long.

The Formative Years

We know that what happens in utero, as well as to newborns in their first months, can have significant health implications: This is no revelation. But more and more studies are telling us how these early inputs, both obvious and not so obvious, influence the risk of allergy and asthma. This gives us some ideas about what we might do early on to change behavior or environment, and to potentially halt the development of disease altogether in the child. As one study put it, "Allergy prevention starts *before* conception: [due to mother-to-fetus] transfer of tolerance, [which] protects against the development of asthma." For new parents, allergy awareness and prevention ought to begin during pregnancy and early in the child's life, the researchers noted, because exposures from the environment impact disease risk.

PREGNANCY

Some researchers have recently explored the relationship between different birth delivery methods and allergy. In a large Danish study, an association was observed (but cause and effect was not proven) between cesarean sections and the child's development of various immune-based conditions, such as asthma and allergies. Other studies have looked at a possible association between C-section and the risk of allergic disorders in children. In 2016, a report suggested that babies delivered by C-section had an increased risk of developing food allergies early in life. At this point, the significance and/or causative role of delivery method have yet to be identified. And I would caution a look at a 2012 Swedish study, which did not support the conclusion that C-section itself explains an increased likelihood of the offspring developing asthma: The researchers observed that multiple factors are responsible for the need for, and type of, C-section—such as emergency—for each delivering mother, including the health of the mother and baby; these considerations may render any association with heightened allergy risk tenuous, at best.

Another proposed risk factor may come off as more surprising (or maybe not): Being born during pollen season heightened the risk of developing allergies and/or eczema. Yet there, too, we should not jump to conclusions (nor do the researchers). Likely there are other mechanisms involved in this finding.

Another study found that for children in families with an allergy history, those who had exposure to a pet dog *before birth*—i.e., the mother was exposed to the pet—were significantly less likely to have eczema and/or wheezing by age three. (Exposure to the dog at or after birth also had a positive impact, though less pronounced.) There is no satisfactory explanation yet for this finding.

A couple of results that likely *won't* surprise you: Among various risk factors for seasonal and indoor allergies—family history of allergic disease; being firstborn—maternal smoking exposure in the first year of life is a powerful one. Certainly, that's a behavioral/environmental modification that is possible to make, to decrease risk, not to mention to decrease the expectant mother's risk of other disease. (Interestingly, active smoking is associated with allergic dermatitis, including eczema, but not allergic rhinitis. Passive smoking is associated with a modest increased risk for both dermatitis and rhinitis.)

The parade of studies about pregnancy and asthma/allergy risk is impressive, if still in relative infancy (pardon the pun). One study from outside the US showed that the use of paracetamol (acetaminophen) by pregnant women correlated with increased asthma risk of the offspring.

Many of these study findings may leave you feeling rather "Okay . . . and then what?" Are you going to time the delivery of your next child to non-pollen season? Refrain from the use of needed medicine? These are not exactly practical behavior modifications. Still, consider this: A study has suggested strong association between receiving allergy injections before or during pregnancy and possible decrease in the likelihood of the child's developing allergies (eczema, allergic rhinitis and/or food allergy).

Don't get *too* excited about the preliminary results referenced above: It's an early observational study, and more long-term data and research will certainly be needed.

I will discuss the hoped-for and actual benefits of immunotherapy/allergy injections later in this chapter.

AVOIDANCE DIETS—MOTHER AND CHILD—AND POSSIBLE PRENATAL INPUT

In my field, one of the hottest research topics is "avoidance diets"—moms not eating certain foods while pregnant, or keeping their young children from eating certain foods, for fear of triggering a reaction (especially in high-risk kids)—or the *opposite* of avoidance diets—namely, exposing children early to certain known allergenic foods, in the hope of reducing the risk of food allergy (ideally, eliminating its development altogether).

The "avoidance diet" crowd seems to be losing: Most recent studies appear to show no marked benefit for the gestating mother or the newborn to avoid highly allergenic foods as a way to prevent the child from developing allergy. In 2008, the American Academy of Pediatrics released guidelines stating that current evidence suggests there is "no benefit" to delaying the introduction of solid foods, past four to six months for preventing allergic outcomes. In the past decade, multiple data have emerged supporting the idea that delaying the introduction of egg, tree nuts, peanut, dairy, shellfish, and fish into the child's diet may actually *increase* allergy risk to those foods. Consult your pediatrician and/or an allergist about when to introduce various foods to your child.

Back in chapter 1, I referenced the study of a set of UK children versus a set of Israeli children, pointing out that the latter group was introduced to peanut at an earlier age and experienced far less prevalence of peanut allergy. What's also potentially compelling about the study: The Israeli mothers "consumed significantly more peanuts during pregnancy" than did pregnant women from the United Kingdom; this pivotal study described an association between higher peanut consumption during the first trimester and lowered chance of a peanut-allergic reaction in the child.

My colleagues who are experts in this area suggest that if you are trying to lower your child's risk of developing food allergy, do not restrict the maternal diet during pregnancy (or lactation). There are no data that suggest that delay has any benefit, and such practice is now outdated. A 2015 clinical trial published in the *New England Journal of Medicine* found that it is safe to introduce peanut-containing foods to the diets of allergic-prone babies in their first year; the study further found that early introduction (compared to delayed introduction) "drastically reduces" their risk of developing peanut allergy when both groups were compared at age five. The study targeted a high-risk group of children, with moderate to severe eczema before four months of life, which demonstrates that while eczema may be associated with food allergy, it does not automatically mean that those who have it also have food allergy, or that they can't handle the early introduction of certain high-risk allergens, such as peanut. These benefits were shown to persist for as long as a year after both groups avoided peanut between ages five and six, with virtually no cases of peanut allergy developing in either group.

General guidelines suggest that foods commonly introduced to the infant should begin at four to six months old. (The World Health Organization [WHO] strongly advocates exclusive breastfeeding for the first six months.) A recent meta-analysis sponsored by the UK Food Standards Agency noted similar protective effects for early egg introduction at four to six months, based on five studies, though no formal recommendations have been made about when, optimally, to introduce egg.

A study of 533 pregnant women who were given either fish oil supplements, olive oil, or no oil during their third trimester found that those children (evaluated in their late teens) whose mothers took the fish oil had a significantly reduced incidence of asthma versus the olive oil cohort. The probability of allergic rhinitis was also lower among adult kids of the fish oil moms versus those of the olive oil moms, but not to a statistically significant degree.

Some researchers have examined the effect of nutrients prenatally, and their ability to modify future atopic disease. They reported that higher levels of vitamin E and zinc were associated with lower risk of wheeze. There is additional data on the possible impact that various minerals consumed during pregnancy might have on the offspring; alas, there is no conclusively positive contribution that we know of yet.

Importantly, we should focus on what kind of dietary philosophy the expectant mother should follow, for her own general good health and her baby's, rather than one vitamin or mineral here or there. In this regard, the Mediterranean diet is broadly recommended. Several studies support that various components of this famously healthy, low-inflammation diet—nuts, vegetables, and fruit, to name three—may have a beneficial impact on asthma, and on seasonal and indoor allergy. Study authors have speculated that a relative lack of allergic symptoms in the group they studied may be attributed to the embrace of the Mediterranean diet. It is believed that this healthy diet may provide a protective effect against asthma and/or allergic conditions. A study published in 2016 in *Pediatric Allergy and Immunology* found that fish intake during pregnancy or infancy may have led to a significant reduction in the risk of eczema and allergic rhinitis in children.

To be conclusive about the impact of these interventions and associations, more large-scale studies of pregnant women and their newborns, with follow-up, are necessary. With these prenatal studies, the results are reported as a change in risk or odds—an indication of probability but far from a defined and certain outcome, and in many cases there are significant caveats that may mean that results do not apply to every patient we see.

BREASTFEEDING AND FORMULA

Breast milk is a crucial food to the developing human. The longer a newborn is breastfed, the better. WHO has very strongly recommended that infants be breastfed exclusively—meaning no other liquid or solid food—for the first six months of life, and this approach is associated with a host of protective benefits ranging from neurocognitive to infectious outcomes. It's suggested that breast milk has an impact on an infant's immune function.

The likelihood that such breastfeeding has a significant impact on food-allergy development long-term, however, is not fully understood or confirmed. Still, because breast milk is hypothesized to help strengthen the newborn's immune system, including the lungs, and because lung infection is an asthma trigger, breastfeeding is considered beneficial in reducing or eliminating the risk of lung infection, which could point to a decreased risk of developing asthma.

So which is it?

Does breastfeeding help with reducing the likelihood of your child developing allergy and asthma—or not? Are the benefits incredibly minor, or are these really exciting findings? My best advice is to stay informed about current guidelines and recommendations, which are constantly evolving. That means having an ongoing dialogue with your pediatrician, ob-gyn physician, and/or allergist. The bottom line is, if you are able to breastfeed your newborn, do so.

AFTER THE BIRTH

It's reported that more and more children need office visits to address their eczema, and that the rate of it has grown over the past several decades. But we have some promising news, and the chance to be proactive: One trial found that applying prescription emollient (moisturizer) to the skin of a newborn at high risk of atopic dermatitis (i.e., a parent or sibling has the condition) through the first thirty-two weeks of her life may help to reduce or prevent the development of the condition. A similar study suggested that reducing the use of detergents and soaps that are excessively drying, in favor of less allergenic moisturizers, may help to optimize the skin barrier early on in life.

It's a great development if the early use of safe topical emollients is found to be meaningfully beneficial, reducing the suffering of infants or young children with unpleasant skin disorders such as eczema. These studies appear not only to "do no harm"; their findings could lead to a universal recommendation, one that benefits a large number of neonates and young children.

Practices for Everyone

While diet and other inputs in the first year of life, or even before birth, can have a magnified impact, that doesn't mean that children, teens, and adults with allergy and asthma cannot turn to alternative, non-medication strategies for possible benefit to their conditions. What follows is a roundup of some whole-body approaches, some of which I recommend to patients, depending on circumstances. None, as far as I can tell, has a negative impact; most of them can have a very positive impact on overall health—physical, psychological, and emotional.

PHYSICAL EXERCISE

Physical exercise contributes all kinds of benefits to one's health, including improved cardiovascular function, greater lung capacity, muscle and bone strength, better skin tone, more restful sleep, and more upbeat and energetic mood. In short, exercise is very strongly associated with quality of life. Exercise focuses appetite, controls weight, and reduces stress. A study reported that physical training, including aerobic-type activities, had improved some breathing measures in those with asthma. Another study looked at the possible benefit of swimming as a training exercise in adolescents and children with asthma: Lung function and cardiovascular fitness improved, a particularly good example of how a healthy habit can improve both one's general fitness and one's disease-specific vulnerability.

Many scientists in this field have lobbied for more research, so we can better understand how to integrate physical training into asthma management. Those with asthma know to take special care when exercising. Warm-up is essential. At least ten to fifteen minutes of non-peak exertion is recommended before peak activity, and periods of intensity might be shorter (though this varies by individual). Those with asthma should take extra caution when exercising in cold weather: Exercise-induced bronchospasm (EIB) reportedly occurs in up to 90 percent of asthmatics.

RELAXATION AND MEDITATION

One study reported that stressful events may precede an eczema outbreak in more than two-thirds of individuals who suffer from the condition. I don't suggest that stress causes eczema, most or even some of the time; indeed, one can very justifiably claim that having eczema or other persistent allergy increases stress, so teasing out one factor from the other is potentially misleading. For now, I'd say that there may be an association between stress and eczema but it's certainly not a prerequisite. Stress may play a role in worsening hives, and one study found stress to be a predisposing factor for half to two-thirds of those with the condition.

Relaxation therapy and other related modalities have been studied in patients with chronic urticaria (hives): Some enjoyed relief from itchiness, some fewer hives. The relaxation response, progressive muscle relaxation, mindfulness meditation, and hypnosis are a few ways you can offset stress. We are unsure precisely how these techniques combat disease or promote healing, but my colleagues and I have had success recommending relaxation techniques, along with pharmacotherapy and other traditional medical approaches, to fight eczema and hives.

BETTER BREATHING AND YOGA

Are there other nonmedication-aided techniques to improve breathing, particularly for the asthmatic? What can the asthmatic do when conventional therapy hasn't helped her to control her condition? Can yoga help?

Breathing techniques can prolong exhalation, among other improvements. Breathing through the nose filters the air. It's better, experts say, for oxygen uptake. The exhale slows the heart rate, and should be longer than the inhale. As anyone who has done breathing exercises knows, this can be a legitimate de-stresser. Conditions like panic disorder may be calmed by this breathing technique: regular, shallow breathing through the nose, at eight to thirteen breaths per minute. Quite a few people get it wrong by deep breathing, which can enable taking in too much air, thus hyperventilation—precisely what a panicked person does *not* want.

Pranayama—a yoga breathing technique—emphasizes deep respiration accompanied by slow exhalation. Buteyko, another breathing technique, is also practiced to improve asthmatic control. In one study of Buteyko, individuals reported fewer asthma symptoms and a reduction in rescue medications. Other studies evaluating Buteyko have not shown benefit, though the technique has a big following in alternative medicine realms.

The truth is that, at least in the credible studies so far, yoga's breathing-specific benefits appear to be small. Still, I find that my patients who use the above techniques on a regular basis appear to have better control of their day-to-day asthma symptoms than those who don't. I acknowledge that the science isn't yet there to support this but if yoga helps give my patients the confidence that they are gaining more control over their stress, as they report to me it does, then that can lead to more control of their asthma.

Another study looked at possible benefits provided by nasal breathing exercises—deep inhale, then exhale through one nostril (with your finger, block the other nostril); hum or make a sound like *om* or *hmm*.

BIOFEEDBACK

Although biofeedback relies more on technology (computers, sensors, wearable devices) than the other practices mentioned in this section, it is at least as concerned as any of them with mindfulness, since it's designed to make you more aware of your physiological functions—heart rate, breathing, muscle contraction, perspiration, body temperature, brainwave activity—that happen without our awareness but are potentially manipulable. One study trained a cohort of asthmatics in controlling their own heart rate to help improve asthma. There were fewer symptoms, lung function improved, and regular medication use was eventually curtailed.

I acknowledge that biofeedback may not work for every asthmatic. Still, for some it may be worth a try.

MASSAGE THERAPY

For one month, parents gave their asthmatic child twenty minutes of massage therapy nightly before bed. The result of this study? There was significant improvement in kids between four and eight years old—an immediate drop in anxiety and cortisol levels and, eventually, better results in pulmonary function tests and in attitude toward asthma. The results for children age nine to fourteen were less pronounced but still measurable: Only one of the quantitative pulmonary measurements got better, but they still reported lower anxiety and better attitude regarding their asthma. I strongly encourage more extensive, controlled testing into the potential benefits of massage.

CHIROPRACTIC MANIPULATION

There are few controlled trials where chiropractic techniques have been used and assessed. In one test of eighty mildly to moderately asthmatic children, each received active spinal manipulation or a simulated technique. When the subjects were evaluated after two months of therapy and then again after four months, the researchers found no meaningful difference in several important criteria (asthma symptoms, morning peak flow rate, airway responsiveness, and more). Another study published by the Cochrane Analysis Group found insufficient evidence to support or dispute the use of manual therapy techniques in asthma; one small trial (the data are yet to be confirmed) found that massage therapy correlated with significant differences in lung function.

AYURVEDIC MEDICINE

Ayurveda is dedicated to the promotion of health more than it is to disease management. Hindu healers encouraged the use of such therapies as yoga, meditation, breathing exercises, and herbal preparations. Some of these herbs are used also in traditional Chinese medicine.

ACUPUNCTURE

Can acupuncture have a meaningful impact on asthma or allergy?

Right now, we don't know. Some of the studies reporting positive outcomes have largely been uncontrolled and randomized trials. They have not produced clinically significant results. The inconclusive nature of some of the latter trials (variation in trial design, incomplete information, small sample size) suggests that bigger, more well-designed trials are required.

Of the trials I've examined, acupuncture's effect on year-round allergy symptoms showed some modest benefit. One study found that acupuncture was associated with a reduction in nasal symptoms within three weeks of the start of treatment. Another study, of those with seasonal allergies, showed statistical improvement and improved quality in their condition, as well as reduced need for antihistamines. Some of the researchers have suggested that gaining benefit from acupuncture might be more realistic for those with mild allergies rather than more serious ones.

Can a combination of acupuncture plus various Chinese herbs provide real benefit to reducing symptoms for those with seasonal allergy? This is worthy of more exploration.

PHOTOTHERAPY (LIGHT THERAPY, UV THERAPY)

Phototherapy is an often helpful approach to managing eczema and psoriasis and perhaps other skin conditions, especially where itchiness is a predominant complaint, and especially when various treatments such as topical creams and ointments and even antihistamines haven't worked. Phototherapy purports to generate an anti-inflammatory effect, reduce itching, boost vitamin D production, and help the body to fight bacteria.

For those of my patients with moderate to severe atopic dermatitis, I have seen phototherapy improve their itchiness (regardless of cause) and eczema.

It works like this: You're exposed to a special machine that emits narrow-band ultraviolet B (UVB) light (though other forms of light may be used, too). For light therapy to be effective, it requires a commitment of at least two to three treatments a week, for an extended period of time.

There is a risk of skin damage. Several large studies on UVB light therapy have not found a link, thankfully, to cancer; a recent Finnish study reached the same conclusion. Talk to your prescribing dermatologist about your particular risk factors, and make an informed decision together.

The success rate of phototherapy is notable: In one account, 70 percent of eczema patients reported that their condition had "quieted" well past their exposure to the light treatments.

My experience with patients tells me that phototherapy can help, and some of my dermatologist colleagues have also reported good suc-

A Link That Doesn't Surprise

Anxiety disorders are prevalent among adults, teens, and kids with asthma. Many approaches to reducing the effects of chronic stress on these cohorts are being studied. It's something I'm investigating every day.

cess using this technique to treat a variety of allergic and non-allergic skin conditions.

SLEEP WELLNESS

The benefits of sufficient, continuous, unstressed sleep, as with physical exercise, are beyond discussion. Good sleep—in quantity and quality—is associated with improved health. At least one study has shown that sleep disturbances are associated with asthma-related symptoms.

It's the chicken-and-egg question: Those individuals with poor control of their nasal allergies and associated congestion are likelier to sleep less well, and not enjoy that great, high-quality REM-associated sleep, and are therefore likelier to complain of daytime fatigue and drowsiness. Or does their lack of sleep make them more vulnerable to allergy? Does their overall fitness set them up for more, and more severe and prolonged, allergy symptoms?

PSYCHOTHERAPY

Cognitive behavioral therapy, supportive counseling, talk therapy—these approaches may all be worth trying, particularly in dealing with skin problems that have resisted all traditional medical solutions.

Immunotherapy

Perhaps the most exciting new development in allergy treatment has been allergen immunotherapy, or AIT, sometimes known as desensitization. The allergen is gradually introduced to the patient (adult or child), creating an immune effect and thus (one hopes) a reduction in symptoms and a halt to the progression of allergy, which can mean a reduction in medication. In short, allergen immunotherapy alters the immune response, enabling long-term tolerance.

For now, it is the best potential way to reduce or even stop allergy symptoms.

Several studies have found allergen immunotherapy to be effective for most properly selected individuals, and it's a universally accepted, proven treatment for allergic rhinitis, allergic rhinoconjunctivitis, allergic asthma and stinging insect allergy. Immunotherapy has been shown to reduce asthma symptoms and use of asthma medications, as well as lessen "irritability" within the lungs. Several studies have reviewed the ability of allergen immunotherapy to help prevent or reduce asthma from developing in children with allergic rhinitis.

Allergy injection immunotherapy, or subcutaneous immunotherapy (SCIT), is the standard treatment that has been used for decades and has an excellent long-term track record of providing significant reduction in allergy symptoms. When administered via shot, immunotherapy is deemed very safe but needs to be done in an allergist's office. (Injections come with a small risk of serious side effects, and, obviously, are less convenient to administer than oral medication.)

What's especially new and exciting: sublingual immunotherapy (SLIT) allergy tablets, which have been approved only recently for use in the United States. The tablets are considered safer than SCIT, and do not need to be given in a doctor's office. The most common adverse side effect of SLIT is localized and oral—swelling, irritation and itchiness of the mouth, throat, and/or lips—which tend to subside within days to a few weeks.

Immunotherapy works particularly well on those with significant sensitization to house dust mite: In one study, patients with asthma and house dust mite (HDM) allergy were given either a placebo or sublingual tablet containing HDM extract. (HDM tablets are not yet approved or available in the US.) And more allergens, such as cat dander, are being targeted for treatment by sublingual tablets.

Until fairly recently, the sole strategies to deal with food allergies were avoidance and vigilance. In many cases, despite one's diligence reading labels and being aware of potential inadvertent exposures, it is difficult to prevent some amount of the food allergen making its way into one's meal, especially when eating out. Immunotherapy has been used on those who are food-allergic but its effectiveness there is still to be determined. The premise: You're fed increasing amounts of an allergenic food, which usually has been baked or heated so that the proteins causing the allergy have been broken down (denatured); or an experimental skin patch is swabbed with the food allergen. A recent clinical trial looked at the benefit of giving very small, controlled amounts of egg to egg-allergic children, so that they could develop a tolerance that was sustainable, and would eventually experience reduced or even no allergic reaction. The effect appears to have been lasting, even long after the oral immunotherapy trial was over; that is, many of the children were still able to safely tolerate a partial serving of egg. (The participants needed to continue their daily amount of egg, even after the supervised trial ended.)

Many parents are desperate to have their children receive oral immunotherapy for their food allergies. Note, however, that it is not a cure; many children experience side effects, including allergic reactions; and most trials have excluded children with a history of anaphylaxis. As new research emerges, continue to discuss options with your child's allergist.

Other Steps Forward

Significant advancements in allergy and asthma care are not reserved for treatment: Better diagnosis is happening, too. We allergists are increasingly using tests that are getting not only more accurate but also more specific. For example, we look for immune reactions to proteins specific to particular substances, and can make distinctions between those with peanut allergy and those with pollen allergy; not so long ago, our tests could not make that sort of differentiation, since the available tests assessed only for allergic reactions to proteins found in both.

BETTER MONITORING

The steps you can take to improve conditions are not necessarily radical.

Some believe that the single most important behavior an allergy or asthma sufferer can embrace is simply to increase the number of visits to the doctor. This can

- improve how well you follow standard therapy (for example, get more regular updates on your condition, such as optimizing your technique of using an inhaler medication)
- establish a better doctor-patient relationship, which provides comfort
- embrace potentially beneficial alternative techniques

At my offices, my team and I do all we can to make each and every patient feel heard, individual, tended to. In other words, it's a patient-centered approach. We explain things at each step. We give printed results of all allergy tests. If a first set of tests doesn't tell us what we need to know, we try a different test. We explain things again because we know it's often hard to take in all the information, from diagnosis to treatment options. We outline the short-term recommendations, then distinguish between those and longer-term remedies. By being thorough, deliberate, and clear, we empower the patient to make informed choices about her course of treatment. By advocating continuity of care, we can properly advise her through all four seasons. We want her to walk out of the office feeling as if there's a way forward, and a plan to get there.

The idea of more frequent doctor visits is not the only nonrevolutionary approach to potentially better treatment: More continuous and/ or intermittent monitoring is recommended as well. As allergy and asthma sufferers well know, a big key to disease management is discipline. One slip can mean unwanted symptoms and a disruption in life plans; it can mean a severe attack. So it's crucial to make sure that you are taking medications when you should; getting allergy shots when you should; staying prepared at all times for emergencies we hope will not come. Allergy and asthma care, especially for those who suffer the moderate to severe version, can be exhausting.

There are new monitoring tools to help you to do this—mobile apps, mobile health devices, and data management software. Here are a couple of new devices that help to improve asthma management:

The Veta is a smart case consisting of a reusable, wearable transparent carrier (plastic case and smart cap) containing various sensors, and a push button to be used in case of emergencies. The wireless connection enables it to link up with the app on a smartphone, iPad, and various tablets. It can help to track the status (activated by pulling off its cap) and/or location of an epinephrine auto-injector with its Find Me feature.

Another device, ADAMM (Automated Device for Asthma Monitoring and Management), was designed for the early detection of asthma: It tracks a number of typical asthma symptoms—cough, heart rate, respiratory rate—so that it may alert you to potential signs of a breathing problem. It can also record when an inhaler is used and provide reminders about your asthma action plan and needed therapies. It can communicate with a website and/or smartphone app, and with your asthma specialist, too.

The above suggestions—better monitoring, better relations with your medical team—represent a very solid form of tertiary prevention, perhaps even secondary prevention, keeping symptoms from getting worse and, at times, cutting off symptom development before it can really get going.

Next Generation

The more our environments and chemical inputs change, the more we need to ask new questions about how we will be affected by allergy and how we will respond. What will be the effect of e-cigarettes, for instance, especially since their liquid flavorings have been evaluated for safety only when consumed orally, not for when they're inhaled?

Does a study by researchers at MIT and the National University of Singapore looking into how house dust mites cause damage to DNA that could prove fatal to lung cells (if one's DNA reparation capacity is compromised) tell us something about the dangers of allergy more profound than what we so far know is true?

Is it true that certain biologics (injectable medicines) can treat moderate to severe asthma? Yes: Along with the use of appropriate asthma medications, this is a promising way to improve asthma management, and studies have shown that the therapy can reduce symptoms and emergency visits, and improve day-to-day quality of life.

It's a new world.

We know so much more about allergy than we did twenty or even ten years ago—yet there are still great mysteries about it yet to be unlocked. There are many theories out there. Are they true? Will they be debunked?

If they're true, are they meaningful?

An esteemed colleague, the pediatric allergist Dr. Mitchell Grayson, has made some intriguing observations: He wonders if and how our mental state plays a crucial role in *how* we experience allergy symptoms. After all, in many allergy studies, the placebo effect produces clinically significant results. And consider this: If it's true that older people tend to have less allergy at least partly because their immune systems react less to allergens, and if it's perhaps true that some women in late-stage pregnancy, as well as those on immunity-suppressing medication, have fewer allergy symptoms (and they *are* true), then maybe it's not so radical to suggest that our responses are a combination of our own particular genetic/physiological makeup; other biochemical influences, including age; our environment and exposure to triggers; and our engagement in life, including mood.

What does all that mean for the allergy sufferer, right now?

As mentioned throughout this book, conventional medicines can provide relief—often medications that are available over the counter, at your local drugstore, ranging from Benadryl to Zyrtec to Claritin. And conventional medicine can also help in longer relief, including nasal steroids and antihistamine sprays.

It's true that conventional therapies do not always provide sufficient relief for all patients. Side effects can sometimes be concerning, particularly in children. With food allergy, no cure exists. Yet we understand the basic principles of allergy treatment: avoidance, environmental modification, pharmacotherapy, and immunotherapy, perhaps the best current option, for many sufferers, for long-term relief and/or remission. Skin patches, a potential form of therapy for the management of food allergies and other conditions, could be on the horizon very soon.

If you were my patient and my team and I were evaluating your allergy condition and options, it would be important for us to understand not merely what the results of, say, your blood test tell us, but also how you want to live your life and what choices you're willing to make. To look at the bigger picture, we need to take a more integrative approach. Ideally, this approach is individualized for you and your condition and where you are in your life. This approach should consider your overall health and your overall goals, not just symptom management. Your new allergy solution should be proactive—demanding much of you. It should be collaborative—so that you feel as if you have support, and a foundation of expertise to call on when needed.

Many answers surrounding allergy remain elusive, but the single most important piece of advice I can impart is that you, the allergy sufferer and health consumer, must stay informed. You needn't know more about your condition than your health provider. But for a collaboration to succeed, you must be fully engaged as you choose the best possible path to the best possible health—whether that means managing symptoms, working to prevent future outbreaks, mediating your home environment, or changing behaviors and diet to shore yourself up and improve your general fitness.

Here's one of the most common questions I get:

Will we one day arrive at an actual cure?

It's a question I can't answer, of course. However, for the distressed patients I see every week in my office, and whose conditions are usually caused by a multitude of factors, and whose situation presents a multitude of questions: For them—for you—I'm happy to say, there is always a solution.

Acknowledgments

Many years ago I had the idea to write a comprehensive book for consumers on allergy because there was nothing quite like it on the market. I'm thrilled that I've finally been able to turn that dream into a reality.

This book would not have happened without the contributions of so many people, in so many capacities.

Many of my esteemed colleagues and friends have given generously of their time and expertise in reviewing and critiquing the chapters related to their specialties. This book benefits immeasurably from their feedback. First and foremost, I would like to thank Dr. Mitchell Grayson, who read though the entire manuscript, going above and beyond with his guidance and constructive comments. I would also like to thank my many colleagues who reviewed one or more chapters for accuracy and accessibility: botanist Dr. Richard Lankow; horticulturist Thomas Ogren; ophthalmologist Dr. Robert Latkany; allergists Dr. David Stukus, Dr. Matthew Greenhawt, Dr. Michael Land, Dr. David Khan, Dr. David Golden, Dr. Maria Castells, and Dr. Gary Gross; allergist and dermatologist Dr. Luz Fonacier; otolaryngologists Dr. Stefan Kieserman, Dr. William Reischacher, Dr. Thomas Romo, III, and Dr. Michael Burnett; neuroscientist Dr. Gregory Ball; and dermatologists

Dr. Doris Day, Dr. Roy Seidenberg, Dr. Anat Lebow, and Dr. Bobby Buka. I would also like to thank all of my staff and colleagues at Allergy & Asthma Care of New York, who have provided ongoing support to me in this endeavor and from whom I have had the opportunity to learn. It truly took a village (of experts) to make this book come about.

I would like to thank my wife, Gail, and my sons, Shawn and Dylan, for encouraging me throughout this endeavor, being my sounding board, tolerating my nonstop work on this project, and lending assistance when deadlines loomed. I would like to thank my literary agent, Beth Vesel, and her assistant, Brita Lundberg, as well as my outstanding collaborator and writing partner, Andrew Postman, without whom this book would not exist. I would also like to thank the diligent team at Penguin Random House, including publishers Adrian Zackheim and Megan Newman, and my editor, Brianna Flaherty, for their guidance all the way to the finish line.

I hope that readers of this book will find answers for their allergy conundrums within these pages, and that these answers can offer a path to meaningfully better health and outlook.

Notes

■

Chapter 1: Trigger Happy

PAGE 3 **These days, spring springs:** Cheryl Katz, "Summer in March? Warming Climate Alters Europe's Seasons," *National Geographic*, April 4, 2016. http://www.news.nationalgeographic.com/2016/04/160404-climate-change-Europe-early-summer/

PAGE 4 **An estimated 30 percent of Americans:** Richard deShazo and Stephen Kemp, "Allergic Rhinitis: Clinical Manifestations, Epidemiology, and Diagnosis," uptodate.com, October 22, 2014. http://www.uptodate.com/contents/allergic-rhinitis-clinical-manifestations-epidemiology-and-diagnosis

PAGE 4 **a Gallup study:** "2005 Gallup Study of Allergies: Phase II Report."

PAGE 4 **Globally, allergy affects 20 to 40 percent:** *WAO White Book on Allergy.* http://www.worldallergy.org

PAGE 4 **The rate in urban environments:** B. Majkowska-Wojciechowska et al, "Prevalence of Allergy, Patterns of Allergic Sensitization and Allergy Risk Factors in Rural and Urban Children," *Allergy*, 2007, 62: 1044–1050.

PAGE 4 **In the United Kingdom:** "Why is Allergy Increasing?" AllergyUK. https://www.allergyuk.org/why-is-allergy-increasing/why-is-allergy-increasing

PAGE 4 **Between 2001 and 2009:** "Asthma Statistics," American Academy of Allergy, Asthma & Immunology, citing Centers for Disease Control and Prevention, *Vital Signs*, May 2011. http://www.aaaai.org/about-aaaai/newsroom/asthma-statistics

PAGE 4 **The CDC says that food allergy in children rose:** Kristen D. Jackson et al, "Trends in Allergic Conditions Among Children: United States,

1997–2011," Centers for Disease Control, May 2013. http://www.cdc.gov/nchs/products/databriefs/db121.htm

PAGE 4 **The rate of peanut allergy doubled:** "Peanut Allergy," Immune Tolerance Network, 2016. http://www.leapstudy.co.uk/peanut-allergy

PAGE 4 **The European Academy of Allergy:** According to the European Academy of Allergy and Clinical Immunology, as referenced in "Facts and Statistics" at Food Allergy Research & Education (FARE). https://www.foodallergy.org/facts-and-stats

PAGE 4 **Ragweed, the central culprit:** Sabrina Tavernise, "Unraveling the Relationship Between Climate Change and Health," *The New York Times*, July 13, 2015. http://www.nytimes.com/2015/07/14/health/unraveling-the-relationship-between-climate-change-and-health.html

PAGE 4 **Combine this with other environmental troubles:** M. Laaidi et al, "Synergy Between Pollen and Air Chemical Pollutants: The Cross Risks; Air Pollution and Allergens," *Environnement, Risques & Santé*, March 2002, 1 (1): 42–49.

J. Bartra et al, "Air Pollution and Allergens," *Allergol Clin Immunol*, 2007, 17 (Suppl. 2): 3–8.

PAGE 5 **bigger and more potent, too:** "Extreme Allergies and Global Warming," National Wildlife Federation, 2010. http://www.nwf.org/pdf/Reports/NWF_AllergiesFinal.pdf; http://www.ucsusa.org/global_warming/science_and_impacts/impacts/warmer-temperatures-allergies.html#.V9ckkyMrJUM

PAGE 5 **In 1950, the native American elm:** Thomas Leo Ogren, "Allergy-Free New York," *The New York Times*, April 5, 2010. http://www.nytimes.com/2010/04/06/opinion/06ogren.html

PAGE 5 **Says renowned horticulturist and author Tom Ogren:** Thomas Leo Ogren, "The Reasons Behind the Modern Pollen Allergy Epidemic," InnerSelf. http://www.innerself.com/content/component/content/article.html?id=4579

PAGE 5 **Wasps, whose stings can cause allergic reaction:** Jayson Maclean, "Climate Change Means Bugs and Insects Are Arriving Earlier This Spring," *CanTech Letter*, April 22, 2016. http://www.cantechletter.com/2016/04/climate-change-means-bugs-insects-arriving-earlier-spring/

PAGE 5 **Fire ants, mostly a fixture:** Lloyd W. Morrison et al, "Predicted Range Expansion of the Invasive Fire Ant, *Solenopsis invicta*, in the Eastern United States Based on the VEMAP Global Warming Scenario," *Diversity and Distributions*, 2005, 11: 199–204. https://www.ars.usda.gov/arsuserfiles/60360510/publications/Morrison_et_al-2005(M-3988).pdf

PAGE 5 **The mostly tropical triatoma:** Stephen A. Klotz et al, "Kissing Bugs in the United States: Risk for Vector-Borne Disease in Humans," *Environ Health Insights*, 2014, 8 (Suppl. 2): 49–59. https://www.ncbi.nlm.nih.gov/pmc/articles/PMC4264683/

PAGE 5 **Mosquitoes are more prevalent:** Aysha Akhtar, "Why Are We Seeing an Explosion of New Viruses Like Zika?" *Huffington Post*, updated February 1, 2016. http://www.huffingtonpost.com/aysha-akhtar/why-are-we-seeing-an-expl_b_9120490.html

PAGE 5 **chikungunya:** "Chikungunya Virus in the United States," Centers for Disease Control and Prevention, August 10, 2016. http://www.cdc.gov/chikungunya/geo/united-states.html

PAGE 5 **dengue fever:** Kim Knowlton, "Climate Change Threatens Health," nrdc.org, October 13, 2015. https://www.nrdc.org/resources/climate-change-threatens-health

PAGE 5 **Forests are flourishing in the eastern United States:** Sabrina Tavernise, "Unraveling the Relationship Between Climate Change and Health," *The New York Times*, July 13, 2015. http://www.nytimes.com/2015/07/14/health/unraveling-the-relationship-between-climate-change-and-health.html

PAGE 5 **In the last fifteen years, the number of annual Lyme cases in Canada:** Sabrina Tavernise, "Unraveling the Relationship Between Climate Change and Health," *The New York Times*, July 13, 2015. http://www.nytimes.com/2015/07/14/health/unraveling-the-relationship-between-climate-change-and-health.html

PAGE 5 **The Lone Star tick, whose name bespeaks:** "Lone Star Tick Continues to Expand Territory to the North, East," DVM360, June 25, 2013. http://www.veterinarynews.dvm360.com/lone-star-tick-continues-expand-territory-north-east

PAGE 6 **mostly climate change:** K. M. Shea et al, "Climate Change and Allergic Disease," *Journal of Allergy and Clinical Immunology*, 2008, 122 (3): 443-453.

PAGE 6 **people exposed to ozone:** "Sneezing and Wheezing," nrdc.org, May 13, 2015. https://www.nrdc.org/resources/sneezing-and-wheezing

PAGE 6 **A study by Quest Diagnostics:** Cody Fenwick, "Allergy Season: Why It Keeps Getting Worse," Across America Patch, March 26, 2016. http://www.patch.com/us/across-america/allergy-season-why-it-keeps-getting-worse-0

PAGE 6 **meaning more carbon dioxide:** "More CO_2 = More Pollen," Climate Central; Ziska et al, 2000 (chart). https://www.ars.usda.gov/agresearchmag/2009/nov/carbon/

"Rising CO_2, Climate Change, and Public Health: Exploring the Links to Plant Biology," *Environ Health Perspect*, February 2009, 117 (2): 155–158. http://www.ehp.niehs.nih.gov/wp-content/uploads/124/4/ehp.124-A70.alt.pdf

PAGE 7 **the introduction of the mosquito-borne:** Sabrina Tavernise, "Unraveling the Relationship Between Climate Change and Health," *The New York Times*, July 13, 2015. http://www.mobile.nytimes.com/2015/07/14/health/unraveling-the-relationship-between-climate-change-and-health.html

PAGE 7 **According to the Natural Resources Defense Council:** "Toxic Chemicals," nrcd.org. https://www.nrdc.org/issues/toxic-chemicals

PAGE 7 **Liquid flavorings in e-cigarettes:** "Put That in Your e-cigarette and Smoke It, or Should You?" UNC Health Care System, February 15, 2016.

PAGE 7 **up to 15 percent of reactions are:** "Drug Allergy Overview," aaaai.org. http://www.aaaai.org/conditions-and-treatments/allergies/drug-allergy

PAGE 7 **A Bristol, England, study:** Susan Dominus, "The Allergy Prison," *The New York Times*, June 10, 2001. http://www.nytimes.com/2001/06/10/magazine/the-allergy-prison.html

PAGE 8 **A German study found:** Bernd Hölscher et al, "Exposure to Pets and Allergies in Children," *Pediatric Allergy and Immunology*, 2002, 13 (5): 334–341.

C. Braun-Fahrländer et al, "Prevalence of Hay Fever and Allergic Sensitization in Farmers' Children and Their Peers Living in the Same Rural Community," *Clin Exp Allergy*, 1999, 29 (1): 28–34.

PAGE 8 **children raised on farms:** Moises Velazquez-Manoff, "A Cure for the Allergy Epidemic?" *The New York Times*, November 9, 2013. http://www.nytimes.com/2013/11/10/opinion/sunday/a-cure-for-the-allergy-epidemic.html

PAGE 8 **dogs and/or cats were less allergically:** D. R. Ownby and C. C. Johnson, "Exposure to Dogs and Cats in the First Year of Life and Risk of Allergic Sensitivity at 6 to 7 Years of Age," *Journal of the American Medical Association*, 2002, 288 (8): 963–972.

A. B. Becker, "Primary Prevention of Allergy and Asthma Is Possible," *Clin Rev Allergy Immunol*, February 2005, 28 (1): 5-16.

PAGE 8 **A decrease in prevalence:** H. Okada et al, "The 'Hygiene Hypothesis' for Autoimmune and Allergic Diseases: An Update," *Clin Exp Immunol*, April 2010, 160 (1): 1–9.

PAGE 8 **projected to be three in five:** "Urban Population Growth," World Health Organization, 2014. http://www.who.int/gho/urban_health/situation_trends/urban_population_growth_text/en/

PAGE 8 **An American Lung Association:** Q. Zhang et al, "Link Between Environmental Air Pollution and Allergic Asthma: East Meets West," *J. Thorac Dis*, January 2015, 7 (1): 14–22.

http://www.thedailybeast.com/cheats/2016/04/20/calif-has-nation-s-most-polluted-air.html;

http://www.sfchronicle.com/news/us/article/Clean-air-advocates-California-has-nation-s-7259028.php

Notes

PAGE 8 **The majority of trees and shrubs:** Thomas Leo Ogren, "Allergy-Free New York," *The New York Times*, April 5, 2010. http://www.nytimes .com/2010/04/06/opinion/06ogren.html

PAGE 9 **In the United States, allergies are the number six:** "Allergies. What's the Problem?" Centers for Disease Control, February 2, 2011. http://www.cdc .gov/healthcommunication/ToolsTemplates/EntertainmentEd/Tips/Allergies .html

PAGE 10 **Certain substances or behaviors:** Astrid Versluis et al, "Cofactors in Allergic Reactions to Food: Physical Exercise and Alcohol Are the Most Important," *Immunity, Inflammation and Disease*, September 15, 2016. http://www.onlinelibrary.wiley.com/doi/10.1002/iid3.120/full#references

PAGE 10 **atopic dermatitis—eczema:** "Eczema in Children," American College of Allergy Asthma & Immunology. http://www.acaai.org/allergies/who-has -allergies/children-allergies/eczema

PAGE 10 **Another study, this one of children:** Kerry E. Drury et al, "Association Between Atopic Disease and Anemia in U.S. Children," *JAMA Pediatr*, 2016, 170 (1): 29–34. http://www.jamanetwork.com/journals/jamapediatrics/article -abstract/2473738

PAGE 10 **severe allergy:** H. B. Kaiser et al, "Risk Factors in Allergy/Asthma," *Allergy Asthma Proc*, January–February 2004, 25 (1): 7–10. https://www.ncbi .nlm.nih.gov/pubmed/15055554

PAGE 11 **If you develop one allergy:** "Do I Have Chronic Allergies?" WebMD. http://www.webmd.com/allergies/guide/chronic-allergies-causes

PAGE 11 **For example, eczema appears:** T. E. Shaw et al, "Eczema Prevalence in the U.S.: Data from the 2013 National Survey of Children's Health," *J Invest Dermatol*, 2011, 131 (1): 67.
C. Flohr and J. Mann, "New Insights into the Epidemiology of Childhood Atopic Dermatitis," *Allergy*, January 2014, 69 (1): 3–16.

PAGE 11 **Up to 80 percent of them will develop:** L. F. Eichenfield et al, "Atopic Dermatitis and Asthma: Parallels in the Evolution of Treatment," *Pediatrics*, March 2003, 111 (3): 608–616. https://www.ncbi.nlm.nih.gov/ pubmed/12612244

PAGE 11 **Infants with food allergies:** A. Schroeder et al, "Food Allergy is Associated with an Increased Risk of Asthma," *Clin Exp Allergy*, February 2009, 39 (2): 261–270. https://www.ncbi.nlm.nih.gov/pmc/articles/ PMC2922978/

PAGE 11 **Why these changes? Let's take a further step back [whole passage]:** Thomas A. E. Platts-Mills and Scott P. Commins, "Increasing Prevalence of Asthma and Allergic Rhinitis," uptodate.com, September 30, 2011. http:// www.cursoenarm.net/uptodate/contents/mobipreview.htm?39/56/40832

PAGE 12 **average size of the family:** David P. Strachan, "Family Size, Infection and Atopy: The First Decade of the 'Hygiene Hypothesis,'" *Thorax*, 2000, 55 (Suppl. 1): S2–S10.

PAGE 12 **It's the developing world's turn:** Thomas A. E. Platts-Mills and Scott P. Commins, "Increasing Prevalence of Asthma and Allergic Rhinitis," uptodate.com, September 30, 2011. http://www.cursoenarm.net/uptodate/contents/mobipreview.htm?39/56/40832

PAGE 12 **Eczema has achieved much:** K. Thestrup-Pedersen, "Atopic Eczema. What Has Caused the Epidemic in Industrialised Countries and Can Early Intervention Modify the Natural History of Atopic Eczema?" *J Cosmet Dermatol*, July 2003, 2 (3–4): 202–210. https://www.ncbi.nlm.nih.gov/pubmed/17163931

PAGE 12 **are farm children, who on average:** Moises Velazquez-Manoff, "A Cure for the Allergy Epidemic?" *The New York Times*, November 9, 2013. http://www.nytimes.com/2013/11/10/opinion/sunday/a-cure-for-the-allergy-epidemic.html

PAGE 15 **A study led by George Du Toit:** "Early Exposure to Peanuts May Prevent Allergy," *Reuters*, November 7, 2008. http://www.reuters.com/article/us-prevent-allergy-idUSTRE4A66IB20081107
   Viva Sarah Press, "Israel's Top Snack Bamba Prevents Peanut Allergy," *Israel 21C*, February 25, 2015. http://www.israel21c.org/israels-top-snack-bamba-prevents-allergy/

PAGE 15 **One of the study's coauthors:** George Du Toit et al, and Gideon Lack for the LEAP Study Team, "Randomized Trial of Peanut Consumption in Infants at Risk for Peanut Allergy: Leap Study Team," *N Engl J Med*, 2015, 372: 803–813.

PAGE 15 **peanut allergy prevalence:** K. Beyer et al, "Effects of Cooking Methods on Peanut Allergencity," *J Allergy Clin Immunol*, June 2001, 107 (6): 1077–1081. https://www.ncbi.nlm.nih.gov/pubmed/11398088

PAGE 16 **In 2008, a report by the American Academy of Pediatrics:** J. A. Boyce et al, "Guidelines for the Diagnosis and Management of Food Allergy in the United States: Report of the NIAID-Sponsored Expert Panel," *J Allergy Clin Immunol*, 2010, 126 (6): 1105–1118. http://www.todaysdietitian.com/newarchives/030413p14.shtml

PAGE 16 **A number of pediatric societies:** Robert S. Zeiger, "Food Allergen Avoidance in the Prevention of Food Allergy in Infants and Children," *Pediatrics*, 2003, 111: 1662–1671.

PAGE 16 **Such dietary avoidance:** "Eczema in Children," American College of Allergy Asthma & Immunology. http://www.acaai.org/allergies/who-has-allergies/children-allergies/eczema

PAGE 16 **food allergy risk to siblings:** R. S. Gupta et al, "Food Allergy Sensitization and Presentation in Siblings of Food Allergic Children," *The*

Journal of Allergy and Clinical Immunology: In Practice, September–October 2016, 4 (5): 956–962.

PAGE 22 **the prevalence of peanut allergy:** A. L. Lee et al, "Food Allergy in Asia: How Does It Compare?" *Asia Pac Allergy*, January 2013, 3 (1): 3–14.

Chapter 2: Defining the Terms, Diagnosing the Problem

PAGE 26 **About 70 percent:** R. J. Kurukulaaratchy et al, "The Influence of Gender and Atopy on the Natural History of Rhinitis in the First 18 Years of Life," *Clin Exp Allergy*, June 2011, 41 (6): 851–859; as referenced in "The Allergy Report" (2000), American Academy of Allergy, Asthma & Immunology. http://www.aaaai.org

PAGE 26 **twice as prevalent as boys:** Joseph Nordqvist, "Hay Fever: Symptoms, Diagnosis and Treatments," *Medical News Today*, June 19, 2015. http://www.medicalnewstoday.com/articles/160665.php

PAGE 26 **Some studies estimate:** Philip L. Lieberman, "Biphasic and Protracted Anaphylaxis." *J Allergy Clin Immunol*, 2011, 78.

PAGE 28 **boys with ADHD are more commonly:** Eelko Hak at al, "Association of Childhood Attention-Deficit/Hyperactivity Disorder with Atopic Diseases and Skin Infections?" *Annals of Allergy, Asthma & Immunology*, August 2013.

PAGE 28 **Of the many kids and teens I see who have ADHD:** Richard deShazo and Stephen Kemp, "Allergic Rhinitis: Clinical Manifestations, Epidemiology, and Diagnosis," uptodate.com, October 22, 2014.

Michael I. Reiff, ed. *ADHD: A Complete and Authoritative Guide.* American Academy of Pediatrics, 2004.

Thomas E. Brown, ed. *ADHD Comorbidities: Handbook for ADHD Complications in Children and Adults.* American Psychiatric Publishing, Inc, 2009.

Sandra F. Rief. *How to Reach and Teach Children with ADD/ADHD: Practical Techniques, Strategies, and Interventions.* Jossey-Bass Teacher, 2005.

PAGE 29 **exposed through the skin to food allergens:** M. Noti, et al, "Exposure to Food Allergens Through Inflamed Skin Promotes Intestinal Food Allergy Through the Thymic Stromal Lymphopoietin-Basophil Axis," *J Allergy Clin Immunol*, May 2014, 133 (5): 1390–1399, e1-6.

PAGE 30 **Dr. Nicholas Furnham:** Nidhi Tyagi et al, "Comparisons of Allergenic and Metazoan Parasite Proteins: Allergy the Price of Immunity," *PLOS Computational Biology*, 2015, 11 (10): e1004546. https://www.sciencedaily.com/releases/2015/10/151029150304.htm

PAGE 30 **It is not even pinworm:** Maria Yazdanbakhsh et al, "Allergy, Parasites, and the Hygiene Hypothesis," *Science*, 2002, 296: 490–494.

"Allergy and Ascariasis." https://www.web.stanford.edu/class/humbio153/AllergyandAscariasis/Background.html

PAGE 31 **Have more kids:** W. Karamaus and C. Botezan, "Does a Higher Number of Siblings Protect Against the Development of Allergy and Asthma? A Review," *J Epidemiol Community Health*, 2002, 56 (3): 209–217.

PAGE 32 **For another, asthma has risen:** Thomas A. E. Platts-Mills and Scott P. Commins, "Increasing Prevalence of Asthma and Allergic Rhinitis," uptodate.com, September 30, 2011. http://www.cursoenarm.net/uptodate/contents/mobipreview.htm?39/56/40832

PAGE 32 **dishwashing by hand:** Alexandra Sifferling, "Why Washing Dishes by Hand May Lead to Fewer Allergies," *Time*, February 23, 2015. http://www.time.com/3717020/dishwashing-allergies/

PAGE 32 **more associated with dogs:** Timo T. Hugg et al, "Exposure to Animals and the Risk of Allergic Asthma: A Population-Based Cross-Sectional Study in Finnish and Russian Children," *Environ Health*, 2008, 7: 28. https://www.ncbi.nlm.nih.gov/pmc/articles/PMC2430194/

PAGE 32 **Antibiotic overuse:** Bryan Love et al, "Antibiotic Prescription and Food Allergy in Young Children," *Allergy, Asthma & Clinical Immunology*, 2016, 12: 41. https://www.aacijournal.biomedcentral.com/articles/10.1186/s13223-016-0148-7, referencing M. S. Ong et al, "Consequences of Antibiotics and Infections in Infancy: Bugs, Drugs, and Wheezing," *Annals of Allergy, Asthma & Immunology*, 2014. http://www.medpagetoday.com/pediatrics/asthma/45759

PAGE 32 **perhaps even doubling it:** "Antibiotic Use in Infants Linked to Asthma," American College of Chest Physicians, June 12, 2007.

A. L. Kozyrsky et al, "Increased Risk of Childhood Asthma from Antibiotic Use in Early Life," *Chest*, June 2007, 131 (6): 1753–1759.

PAGE 36 **If one parent has/had allergy:** "Allergy Prevention," Auckland Allergy Clinic, October 16, 2006. www.allergyclinic.co.nz/allergy_prevention.aspx

Chapter 3: What Does Prevention Look Like?

PAGE 42 **At a recent seminar, an expert spoke:** http://www.my.clevelandclinic.org/health/diseases_conditions/hic_Asthma_An_Overview/hic_Understanding_Asthma_Triggers/hic_Stress_and_Asthma

PAGE 43 **recent study from the University of British Columbia:** "Air Pollution Exposure During Pregnancy Linked with Asthma Risk," *The University of British Columbia Health News*, February 23, 2016.

PAGE 45 **nearly one-third of all Americans:** "Shingles (Herpes Zoster)," CDC.gov, August 19, 2016. http://www.cdc.gov/shingles/about/overview.html

PAGE 45 **Recent guidelines:** Food Allergy Practice Parameter Update 2014, *J Allergy Clin Immunol*, 2014, 134: 1016–1025.

PAGE 45 **an important National Institutes of Health-funded:** George Du Toit et al, and Gideon Lack/LEAP-On Study Team, "Effect of Avoidance on

Peanut Allergy After Early Peanut Consumption," *New England Journal of Medicine*, March 7, 2016.

PAGE 46 **Primary prevention may include:** P. Nair, "Early Interventions with Inhaled Corticosteroids in Asthma: Benefits and Risks," *Curr Opin Pulm Med*, 2011, 17 (1): 6–11.

PAGE 47 **Other examples include:** "Prevention of Allergy and Allergic Asthma," World Health Organization, January 8–9, 2002. http://www.who.int/ respiratory/publications/WHO_NMH_MNC_CRA_03.2.pdf

Chapter 4: Nose and Sinuses, Face, Lung, Eyes: Some Basic Allergies
PAGE 55 **to around 75–80 percent humidity:** S. Musheer Hussain, ed. *Logan Turner's Diseases of the Nose, Throat and Ear: Head and Neck Surgery*. Boca Raton, FL: CRC Press, 2016, p. 9.

PAGE 55 **processing more than fourteen thousand liters:** "Principles of Nasal Irrigation," NeilMed Pharmaceuticals, Inc., April 23, 2010. http://www.neilmed.com/neilmedblog/2010/04/principles-of-nasal -irrigation/

PAGE 55 **report sleep-related problems:** "Allergies and Sleep," National Sleep Foundation, December 2009. https://www.sleepfoundation.org/sleep-topics/ sleep-related-problems/allergic-rhinitis-and-sleep

PAGE 56 **Boy noses and:** Honor Whiteman, "Why Men's Noses are Bigger Than Women's," *Medical News Today*, November 23, 2013. http://www .medicalnewstoday.com/articles/269199.php

PAGE 59 **The Mayo Clinic reports:** "Nonallergic Rhinitis," Mayo Clinic. http://www.mayoclinic.org/diseases-conditions/nonallergic-rhinitis/ symptoms-causes/dxc-20179169

PAGE 60 **National Center for Complementary:** NCCIH.nih.gov

PAGE 61 **Small studies have indicated:** J. A. Bernstein et al, "A Randomized, Double-Blind, Parallel Trial Comparing Capsaicin Nasal Spray with Placebo in Subjects with a Significant Component of Nonallergic Rhinitis," *Ann Allergy Asthma Immunol*, August 2011, 107 (2): 171–178.

PAGE 61 **Longer-term complications may arise:** "Nonallergic Rhinitis," Mayo Clinic, January 26, 2016. http://www.mayoclinic.org/diseases-conditions/ nonallergic-rhinitis/symptoms-causes/dxc-20179169

PAGE 62 **Allergic rhinitis is thought to affect:** Izquierdo-Domínguez et al, "Comparative Analysis of Allergic Rhinitis in Children and Adults," *Curr Allergy Asthma Rep*, April 2013, 13 (2): 142–151.

PAGE 63 **What They Do for You, and How:** "Allergic Rhinitis," Quality Management Program, University of Michigan, October 2013. http://www .med.umich.edu/1info/FHP/practiceguides/allergic/allergic.pdf

PAGE 64 **A number of sources point:** "Chronic Respiratory Diseases," World

Health Organization. http://www.who.int/gard/publications/chronic
_respiratory_diseases.pdf

PAGE 66 **Polyps are twice as common:** "What Are Nasal Polyps?" WebMD,
2014. http://www.webmd.com/allergies/guide/nasal-polyps-symptoms-and
-treatments

PAGE 66 **Nasal polyps can also be:** "Nasal Polyps: Risk factors," Mayo Clinic,
March 8, 2014. http://www.mayoclinic.org/diseases-conditions/nasal-polyps/
basics/risk-factors/con-20023206

PAGE 67 **the connection with nasal allergy hasn't:** "What Are Nasal Polyps?"
WebMD, 2014. http://www.webmd.com/allergies/guide/nasal-polyps
-symptoms-and-treatments

PAGE 67 **As much as 10 to 15 percent:** Pnina Weiss and Kenneth Rundell,
"Imitators of Exercise-Induced Bronchoconstriction," *Allergy, Asthma &
Clinical Immunology*, 2009. https://www.aacijournal.biomedcentral.com/
articles/10.1186/1710-1492-5-7

PAGE 68 **In allergic asthma, when your immune system:** Jenna Murdoch and
Clare Lloyd, "Chronic Inflammaton and Asthma," *Mutat Res*, August 7,
2010, 690 (1–2): 24–39. https://www.ncbi.nlm.nih.gov/pmc/articles/
PMC2923754

PAGE 69 **For some people, food and drug:** "Allergies and Asthma: They
Often Occur Together," Mayo Clinic, February 13, 2016. http://www
.mayoclinic.org/diseases-conditions/asthma/in-depth/allergies-and-asthma/
art-20047458

  "Medications May Trigger Asthma Symptoms," aaaai.org. http://www
.aaaai.org/conditions-and-treatments/library/asthma-library/medications-that
-can-trigger-asthma-symptoms

PAGE 69 **Roughly half of all adults:** "Prevention of Allergy and Allergic
Asthma," World Health Organization, January 8–9, 2002. http://www
.who.int/respiratory/publications/WHO_NMH_MNC_CRA_03.2.pdf

PAGE 69 **80 to 90 percent of asthmatic kids:** K. C. Barnes, "Genetic Studies of
the Etiology of Asthma," *Proc Am Thorac Soc*, May 2011, 8 (2): 143–148.

  J. Kiley et al, "Asthma Phenotypes," *Curr Opin Pulm Med*, January 2007,
13 (1): 19–23.

  R. A. Mathias, "Introduction to Genetics and Genomics in Asthma:
Genetics of Asthma," *Adv Exp Med Biol*, 2014, 795: 125–155.

  J. W. Mims, "Asthma: Definitions and Pathophysiology," *Int Forum
Allergy Rhinol*, September 2015, 5 (Suppl. 1): S2–S6.

PAGE 69 **by age forty:** "The Allergy Report," 2000, American Academy of
Allergy, Asthma & Immunology. http://www.aaaai.org

PAGE 69 **More women die from it:** "Asthma," CDC, May 3, 2016. http://www
.cdc.gov/asthma

PAGE 69 **hormone replacement therapy:** Heather Hatfield, "The Impact of Female Hormones on Asthma," WebMD. http://www.webmd.com/asthma/features/asthma-women

European Lung Foundation, "HRT Therapy Appears to Increase Risk of Hospitalization from Severe Asthma Attacks, Research Suggests," *ScienceDaily*, September 27, 2011.

PAGE 70 **If you have hay fever or other allergies:** "Asthma Risk Factors," American Lung Association.

PAGE 70 **Ask your asthma specialist:** "Asthma Control Test," asthma.com, 2015. http://www.asthma.com/additional-resources/asthma-control-test.html

PAGE 70 **Children often outgrow:** "Asthma Risk Factors," WebMD, 2016. http://www.webmd.com/asthma/guide/asthma-risk-factors

PAGE 71 **Long-term controller medication:** National Asthma Education and Prevention Program, "Expert Panel Report III: Guidelines for the Diagnosis and Management of Asthma," Bethesda, MD: National Heart, Lung, and Blood Institute, 2007. http://www.nhlbi.nih.gov/health-pro/resources/lung/naci/discover/corticosteriods.htm, www.nhlbi.nih.gov/guidelines/asthma/asthgdln.htm

PAGE 72 **There's clear evidence that:** Diarmuid M. McNicholl et al, "Omalizumab: The Evidence for Its Place in the Treatment of Allergic Asthma," *Core Evid*, June 2008, 3 (1): 55–66.

PAGE 72 **Allergy shots (immunotherapy):** M. J. Abramson et al, "Injection Allergen Immunotherapy for Asthma," Cochrane Database of Systematic Reviews, 2010, 8, article number CD001186.

P. S. Norman, "Immunotherapy: 1999–2004," *J Allergy Clin Immunol*, 2004, 113 (6): 1013.

PAGE 73 **Incredibly, reports indicate that:** "Asthma Self-Management Education by Age, U.S., 2008," National Health Interview Survey, as it appears on the CDC website. http://www.cdc.gov/vitalsigns/asthma/

PAGE 74 **thought to occur in 2 percent:** Gwen Smith, "Risk of Anaphylaxis Now 1 in 50 People," AllergicLiving, http://www.allergicliving.com/2013/11/19/risk-of-anaphylaxis-now-1-in-50-people/

PAGE 74 **up to 8 percent:** Robert Wood et al, "Anaphylaxis in America: The Prevalence and Characteristics of Anaphylaxis in the United States," *J Allergy Clin Immunol*, February 2014. http://www.aafa.org/media/Anaphylaxis-in-America-JACI-Article-2014.pdf

PAGE 74 **Though these are rare, anaphylaxis:** Robert Wood et al, "Anaphylaxis in America: The Prevalence and Characteristics of Anaphylaxis in the United States," *J Allergy Clin Immunol*, February 2014. http://www.aafa.org/media/Anaphylaxis-in-America-JACI-Article-2014.pdf

PAGE 75 **Those with allergies or asthma:** "Anaphylaxis Risk Factors," Mayo Clinic, January 16, 2013. http://www.mayoclinic.org/diseases-conditions/anaphylaxis/basics/risk-factors/con-20014324

PAGE 76 **50 million mast cells:** J. Y. Niederkorn, ed., *Immune Response and the Eye*. Basel: Karger, 2007.

PAGE 76 **Five of every six people:** "2005 Gallup Study of Allergies: Phase II Report."

PAGE 76 **An much as 20 percent:** E. L. Bolling, "Is It Dry Eye, Allergy or Both?" *Review of Optometry*, September 2012. http://www.healthywomen.org/condition/ocular-allergies

PAGE 76 **half of all women said that eye-impacted allergies:** "Eye Allergies Disrupt Daily Activities, Impact Performance and Appearance," Johnson & Johnson, March 14, 2012. https://www.jnj.com/media-center/press-releases/eye-allergies-disrupt-daily-activities-impact-performance-and-appearance-survey-shows

PAGE 76 **For treating eye allergy:** Warner Carr et al, "Treating Allergic Conjunctivitis: A Once-Daily Medication That Provides 24-Hour Symptom Relief," *Allergy Rhinol* (Providence), Summer 2016, 7 (2): e107–e114. http://www.uptodate.com/contents/allergic-conjunctivitis-management#H12817219

PAGE 78 **GPC is a more extreme form:** "Giant Papillary Conjunctivitis (GPC)," DoveMed, June 26, 2016. http://www.dovemed.com/giant-papillary-conjunctivitis-gpc/

PAGE 79 **This condition tends to worsen:** "Atopic Keratoconjunctivitis," DoveMed, March 15, 2016. http://www.dovemed.com/atopic-kerato conjunctivitis-akc/

PAGE 79 **three-quarters of those who have it:** "Eye Allergy," acaai.org, 2014. http://www.acaai.org/allergies/types/eye-allergies

PAGE 79 **Dry eye may be triggered:** Mohammad-Ali Javadi and Sepehr Feizi, "Dry Eye Syndrome," *J Ophthalmic Vis Res*, July 2011, 6 (3): 192–198. https://www.ncbi.nlm.nih.gov/pmc/articles/PMC3306104/

PAGE 81 **Allergies may contribute to blepharitis:** Cheryl Guttman Krader, "Research Sheds Light on Posterior Blepharitis," *Ophthalmology Times*, March 15, 2010. http://www.ophthalmologytimes.modernmedicine.com/ophthalmologytimes/news/modernmedicine/modern-medicine-feature-articles/research-sheds-light-posteri

Chapter 5: Outdoor and Seasonal Allergies

PAGE 83 **Roughly 20 percent of allergy sufferers:** "Allergies, Nasal In-Depth Report," *The New York Times*, 2008. http://www.nytimes.com/health/guides/disease/allergic-rhinitis/print.html

Notes

PAGE 84 **Researchers explain the nature of the problem:** Betul Sin and Alkis Togias, "Pathophysiology of Allergic and Nonallergic Rhinitis," Proceedings of the American Thoracic Society, 2011, 8 (1): 106–114.

PAGE 84 **nasal symptoms at the end of pollen season:** J. R. Bacon et al, "Priming of the Nasal Mucosa by Ragweed Extract or by an Irritant (Ammonia)," from the Division of Allergy, Department of Internal Medicine, University of Michigan Medical School, Ann Arbor, *JACI*, February 1981, 67 (2): 11–116.

PAGE 84 **from the University of Chicago:** University of Chicago Medical Center, "Steroids More Effective Than Antihistamines When Used as Needed for Allergies," *Science Daily*, November 27, 2001. https://www .sciencedaily.com/releases/2001/11/011127004650.htm

PAGE 84 **it can take approximately three seasons:** Richard deShazo and Stephen Kemp, "Allergic Rhinitis: Clinical Manifestations, Epidemiology, and Diagnosis," uptodate.com, October 22, 2014.

PAGE 84 **Due to climate change:** "Warming Temperatures Drive Up Pollen Production and Allergies," Union of Concerned Scientists. http://www .ucsusa.org/global_warming/science_and_impacts/impacts/warmer -temperatures-allergies.html#.V9ckkyMrJUM

PAGE 87 **10,000 feet in the air:** "Pollen and Environmental Allergies," New York Allergy & Sinus Centers, http://www.advancedallergyny.com/pollen _allergies.php

PAGE 88 **There are over one thousand:** "Pollen Allergy: What Is It?" medicinenet.com. http://www.medicinenet.com/script/main/art.asp

PAGE 88 **In much of Texas:** "ImmunoCAP Tree Pollens Allergens," ThermoFisher Scientific, 2008. http://www.texasmonthly.com/the-culture/ texas-primer-cedar-fever/

PAGE 88 **Some Southwestern cities:** Pauline Arrillaga, "Arizona Desert Is No Oasis for Allergy Victims," *Los Angeles Times*, October 10, 1999. http://www .articles.latimes.com/1999/oct/10/news/mn-20913

PAGE 90 **[MAP]:** National Allergy Bureau, American Academy of Allergy, Asthma & Immunology, prepared by and courtesy of Richard Lankow, PhD, Director, Medical and Scientific Affairs Education, Aspen Bioscience LLC.

PAGE 91 **[MAP]:** USDA Plants Database, http://www.plants.usda.gov, prepared by and courtesy of Richard Lankow, PhD, Director, Medical and Scientific Affairs Education, Aspen Bioscience LLC

PAGE 92 **Smart Steps:** (From interview with author) Cody Fenwick, "Allergy Sufferers: New Treatments Provide Hope, Relief," Patch.com, March 28, 2016. http://www.patch.com/us/across-america/spring-allergies-new -treatments-old-tips-0

PAGE 92 **An FFP2 dust mask:** The Dust Mask Store. http://www.thedustmask store.com/dust-masks.html

PAGE 94 **a spike in emergency room:** University of Georgia, "Thunderstorms Linked to Asthma Attacks," *Science Daily*, July 2008. https://www .sciencedaily.com/releases/2008/07/080710131424.htm

PAGE 94 **the air in a thunderstorm:** Dr. Annie Arrey-Mensah, "What Is Thunderstorm Asthma?" AAIIMichigan.com. http://www.aaiimichigan.com/ pdfs/Thunderstorm%20Asthma.pdf

PAGE 102 **Sting Operation: Know Your Insects [bulk of passage]:** "Stinging Insect Allergy," American Academy of Allergy, Asthma & Immunology. http://www.aaaai.org/conditions-and-treatments/library/allergy-library/ stinging-insect-allergy

PAGE 105 **Venom immunotherapy is currently:** D. B. Golden et al, "Regimens of Hymenoptera Venom Immunotherapy," *Ann Intern Med*, 1980, 92 (5): 620.

PAGE 105 **This condition, termed Skeeter syndrome:** F. E. Simons and Z. Peng, "Skeeter Syndrome," *J Allergy Clin Immunol*, 1999, 104 (3, part 1): 705.

PAGE 109 **And high elevations:** F. Spieksma et al, "High Altitude and House Dust Mites," *Br Med J*, 1971, 1: 82–84.

Chapter 6: Indoor Environment

PAGE 112 **On average, we spend 80 to 90 percent:** https://www.epa.gov/indoor -air-quality-iaq/inside-story-guide-indoor-air-quality

PAGE 112 **One study found that more than half:** P. J. Vojta et al, "The National Survey of Lead and Allergens in Housing," *Environmental Health Perspectives*, May 2002, 110 (5): 527–532.

PAGE 113 **By 2030:** "Urban Population Growth," World Health Organization, 2014. http://www.who.int/gho/urban_health/situation_trends/urban _population_growth_text/en/

PAGE 113 **Some researchers believe:** G. D'Amato, "Environmental Urban Factors (Air Pollution and Allergens) and the Rising Trends in Allergic Respiratory Diseases," *Allergy*, 2002, 57 (Suppl. 72): 30–33.

PAGE 113 **A 2012 European study:** Chiara Ziello, "Changes to Airborne Pollen Counts Across Europe," *PLoS ONE*, April 13, 2012, 7 (4): e34076.

PAGE 113 **Young children, from infants:** H. Y. Kim et al, "Determinants of Sensitization to Allergen in Infants and Young Children," *Korean J Pediatrics*, May 2014, 57 (5): 205–210.

PAGE 113 **The critical period for allergen sensitization:** P. G. Holt et al, "The Role of Allergy in the Development of Asthma," *Nature*, 1999, 402 (Suppl.): B12–B17.

PAGE 113 **Sensitization to the major allergen:** Elizabeth Matsui et al, "Asthma in the Inner City and the Indoor Environment," *Immunol Allergy Clin N Am*, 2008. http://www.hopkinsmedicine.org/pulmonary/research/adherence _research/document_links/matsui_hansel_mccormack.pdf

PAGE 114 **Yet these new building designs:** D. Norback et al, "Indoor Air Quality and Personal Factors Related to the Sick Building Syndrome," *Scand J Work Environ Health*, 1990, 16: 121–128.

PAGE 114 **those who live on farms:** Moises Velazquez-Manoff, "A Cure for the Allergy Epidemic?" *The New York Times*, November 9, 2013. http://www .nytimes.com/2013/11/10/opinion/sunday/a-cure-for-the-allergy-epidemic .html

PAGE 115 **That pillow you've used for:** T. J. Kemp et al, "House Dust Mite Allergens in Pillows," *BMJ*, 1996, 313: 91.

   Ohio State University Extension Fact Sheet. http://www.ohioline.ag.ohio -state-edu

PAGE 115 **After fifteen minutes of disturbance:** J. A. Meadows, "Allergy Avoidance—Dust Mites." http://www.medfusion.net/templates/ groups/5766/10074/AllergyAvoidanceDustMites.pdf; J. Portnoy et al, Joint Taskforce on Practice Parameters Workgroup, "Environmental Assessment and Exposure Control of Dust Mites: A Practice Parameter," Ann Allergy Asthma Immunol, December 2013, 111 (6): 465–507.

PAGE 116 **Dust Never Sleeps:** E. J. Popplewell, "The Effect of High-Efficiency and Standard Vacuum Cleaners on Mite, Cat and Dog Allergen Levels and Clinical Progress," *Pediatr Allergy Immunol*, 2000, 11 (3): 142.

PAGE 115 **Because cat and dog allergen:** "Dog Dander," Thermo Scientific, 2012. http://www.phadia.com/fr/5/Produits/ImmunoCAP-Allergens/Epidermals -and-Animal-Proteins/Allergens/Dog-dander/

PAGE 117 **Porous/stuffed toys:** C. F. Chang et al, "Effect of Freezing, Hot Tumble Drying and Washing with Eucalyptus Oil on House Dust Mites in Soft Toys," *Pediatric Allergy Immunology*, 2011, 22: 638–641.

PAGE 118 **HEPA air filters appear to be beneficial:** E. J. Popplewell et al, "The Effect of High-Efficiency and Standard Vacuum Cleaners on Mite, Cat and Dog Allergen Levels and Clinical Progress," *JA Pediatr Allergy Immunol*, 2000, 11 (3): 142.

PAGE 118 **High-efficiency whole house filtration:** J. L. Sublett, "Effectiveness of Air Filters and Air Cleaners in Allergic Respiratory Diseases: A Review of the Recent Literature," *Curr Allergy Asthma Rep*, October 2011, 11 (5): 395–402.

PAGE 118 **Steam-cleaning can kill:** M. J. Colloff et al, "The Use of Domestic Steam Cleaning for the Control of House Dust Mites," *Clin Exp Allergy*, November 1995, 25 (11): 1061–1066.

PAGE 119 **allergy to rodents is more likely:** W. Phipatanakul et al, "Environmental Assessment and Exposure Reduction of Rodents: A Practice Parameter," *Ann Allergy Asthma Immunol*, December 2012, 109 (6): 375–387.

PAGE 119 **In suburban homes:** I. Stelmach et al, "The Prevalence of Mouse Allergen in Inner-City Homes," *Pediatric Allergy and Immunology*, August 2002, 13 (4): 299–302.

PAGE 119 **Worse, the level in inner-city schools:** W. J. Sheehan et al, "Mouse Allergens in Urban Elementary Schools and Homes of Children with Asthma," *Ann Allergy Asthma Immunol*, 2009, 102 (2): 125.

PAGE 119 **Asthma is found at epidemic levels:** W. J. Sheehan et al, "Mouse Allergens in Urban Elementary Schools and Homes in Children with Asthma," *Ann Allergy Asthma Immunol*, February 2009, 102 (2): 125–130.

PAGE 119 **Over time, mice can develop:** Rodenticide Resistance Action Group (RRAG) House Mouse Resistance Guideline, August 15, 2012. http://www.bpca.org.uk/assets/RRAG-Housemouseresistanceguideline1.pdf

PAGE 120 **Researchers can detect cockroach:** W. J. Sheehan et al, "Pest and Allergen Exposure and Abatement in Inner-City Asthma: A Work Group Report of the American Academy of Allergy, Asthma & Immunology, Indoor Allergy/Air Pollution Committee," *J Allergy Clin Immunol*, March 2010, 125 (3): 575–581.

PAGE 120 **As with rodent infestation:** W. J. Sheehan et al, "Pest and Allergen Exposure and Abatement in Inner-City Asthma: A Work Group Report of the AAAAI Indoor Allergy–Air Pollution Committee," *J Allergy Clin Immunol*, 2010, 125: 575–581.

PAGE 120 **Studies have shown an association:** Thomas A. Platts-Mills, "Asthma Severity and Prevalence: An Ongoing Interaction Between Exposure, Hygiene, and Lifestyle," *PLoS Med*, February 2005, 2 (2): e34.

PAGE 120 **Repair leaks immediately:** "Environmental Triggers of Asthma Treatment, Management, and Prevention," from the Agency for Toxic Substances & Disease Registry, an agency of the U.S. Department of Health and Human Services, November 28, 2014. http://www.atsdr.cdc.gov/csem/csem.asp?csem=32&po=9

PAGE 121 **A study in Finland found that a yard:** Wynne Parry, "Backyard Diversity May Stem Allergies," *LiveScience*, May 7, 2012. http://www.livescience.com/20139-microbes-diversity-allergies.html#sthash.hxaNeFDN

PAGE 123 **The ficus (including rubber tree):** Thomas Leo Ogren, *The Allergy-Fighting Garden: Stop Asthma and Allergies with Smart Landscaping*. Potter/TenSpeed/Harmony, 2015.

PAGE 123 **We shed about one-fifth:** "Indoor Air Pollutants and Toxic Materials," Centers for Disease Control, 2006. http://www.cdc.gov/nceh/publications/books/housing/2006_hhm_final_chapter_05.pdf

Notes

PAGE 123 **They're found the world over:** "Indoor Air Pollutants and Toxic Materials," Centers for Disease Control, 2006. http://www.cdc.gov/nceh/publications/books/housing/2006_hhm_final_chapter_05.pdf

PAGE 123 **A link between HDMs:** "Indoor Air Pollutants and Toxic Materials," Centers for Disease Control, 2006. http://www.cdc.gov/nceh/publications/books/housing/2006_hhm_final_chapter_05.pdf

PAGE 123 **When the allergen exceeds:** "Study Shows Simple Steps Can Reduce Dust Mite Allergens in Bedrooms," NIH/National Institute of Environmental Health Sciences, August 7, 2001. https://www.sciencedaily.com/releases/2001/08/010807080452.htm

PAGE 123 **One survey found dust mite:** Arbes et al, "House Dust Mite Allergen in U.S. Beds: A National Survey of Allergens in Housing," *JACI*, 2002, 111 (2).

PAGE 124 **In a 2011 compilation:** "Ranking of Worst Big Cities for Allergies," Quest Diagnostics Health Trends, 2011. http://www.questdiagnostics.com/dms/Images/BodyCopy/Specific_segment_or_topic/Health-Trends/Allergy/Ranking_of_Cities_for_allergies_table

PAGE 125 **"Bedrooms are (ideally) carpet-free":** "Environmental Triggers of Asthma Treatment, Management, and Prevention," from the Agency for Toxic Substances & Disease Registry, an agency of the U.S. Department of Health and Human Services, November 28, 2014. http://www.atsdr.cdc.gov/csem/csem.asp?csem=32&po=9

PAGE 126 **Studies of how to kill dust mites:** A. F. Kalpaklioglu et al, "The Effectiveness of Benzyl Benzoate and Different Chemicals as Acaricides," *Allergy*, 1996, 51: 164–170.

PAGE 126 **A study from Kingston University:** C. Claiborne Ray, "Q&A: Dust Mites No Excuse Not to Make Bed," *The New York Times*, January 19, 2016, D2.

PAGE 126 **recommend air filtration:** K.V. Vannan et al, "Enhancing Indoor Air Quality: The Air Filter Advantage," *Lung India*, September–October 2015, 32 (5): 473–479.

PAGE 127 **Limit the presence of carpets:** T. A. Platts-Mills et al, "Indoor Allergens and Asthma: Report of the Third International Workshop," *J Allergy Clin Immunol*, 1997, 100 (6, part 1): S2.

PAGE 127 **It can take just four months:** P. A. Eggleston and A. Boner, "Improving Indoor Environments: Reducing Allergen Exposures," *J Allergy Clin Immunol*, July 2005, 116 (1): 122–126.

A. Boner et al, "The Role of House Dust Mite Elimination in the Management of Childhood Asthma: An Unresolved Issue," *Allergy*, 2002, 57 (Suppl. 74): 23–31.

PAGE 127 **The greatest concentration of indoor:** Arbes et al, "House Dust Mite

Notes

Allergen in U.S. Beds: A National Survey of Allergens in Housing," *JACI*,2002, 111 (2).

P. J. Vojta, "The National Survey of Lead and Allergens in Housing," *Environmental Health Perspectives,* May 2002, 110 (5): 527–532.

P. M. Salo et al, "Dustborne Alternaria Alternata Antigens in U.S. Homes: Results from the National Survey of Allergens in Housing," *J Allergy Clin Immunol,* September 2005, 116 (3): 623–629.

PAGE 128 **While dry vacuum cleaning:** Fell et al, in a letter in *Lancet,* 1992, 340: 788–789.

PAGE 128 **Allergen levels register higher:** D. Crowther et al, "House Dust Mites and the Built Environment: Literature Review," September 2000.

PAGE 130 **About 85 percent of the contaminants:** "Controlling Pollutants and Sources: Indoor Air Quality Design Tools for Schools," EPA, referencing the International Sanitary Supply Association, August 13, 2016. https://www.epa .gov/iaq-schools/controlling-pollutants-and-sources-indoor-air-quality-design -tools-schools#Entry Mat Barriers

PAGE 131 **Pet ownership is the strongest:** "Pet Allergies," acaai.org. http://www .acaai.org/allergies/types/pet-allergy

PAGE 131 **The levels detected in homes:** Arbes et al, "Dog Allergen (Can f 1) and Cat Allergen (Fel d 1) in U.S. Homes: Results from the National Survey of Lead and Allergens in Housing," *J Allergy Clin Immunol,* 2004, 114: 111–117.

PAGE 131 **Cat allergen is particularly:** P. M. Salo, "Dustborne Alternaria Alternata Antigens in U.S. Homes: Results from the National Survey of Allergens in Housing," *J Allergy Clin Immunol,* September 2005, 116 (3): 623–629.

PAGE 131 **Sleeping on animal fur:** "Sleeping on Animal Fur in Infancy Found to Reduce Risk of Asthma," European Lung Foundation, September 8, 2014. https://www.sciencedaily.com/releases/2014/09/140908083750.htm

PAGE 132 **For allergen levels in carpets:** T. Dybendal and S. Elsayed, "Dust from Carpeted and Smooth Floors. V. Cat. (Fed d 1) and Mite (Der p 1 and Def f 1) Allergen Levels in School Dust," *Clin Exp Allergy,* December 1992, 22 (12): 1100–1106.

R. D. Lewis and P. N. Breysse, "Carpet Properties That Affect the Retention of Cat Allergen," *Ann Allergy Asthma Immunol,* July 2000, 85 (1): 27.

PAGE 132 **One study showed that high:** Wood et al, "A Placebo-Controlled Trial of a HEPA Air Cleaner in the Treatment of Cat Allergy," *Am J Respir Crit Care Med,* July 1998, 158 (1): 115–120.

PAGE 132 **Carpet accumulates cat allergen:** "Managing Pet Allergies,"

healthstatus.com. https://www.healthstatus.com/health_blog/allergies
-asthma-sinus/managing-pet-allergies/

PAGE 132 **Litter boxes may contain:** "Allergens," kittentesting.com, 2005.
http://www.kittentesting.com/allergens.html

PAGE 132 **Cat allergy is more prevalent:** Lindsey Konkel, "Nothing to Sneeze
At: Cats Worse Than Dogs for Allergies," *LiveScience*, July 26, 2012. http://
www.livescience.com/36578-cat-worse-dogs-allergies-pets.html

PAGE 132 **dog allergen (Can f 1) is found:** A.Woodcock and A. Custovic,
"Allergen Avoidance: Does It Work?" *British Medical Bulletin*, 2000, 56 (4):
1071–1086.

PAGE 132 **Frequent dog-washing:** T. Hodson et al, "Washing the Dog Reduces
Allergen Levels, But the Dog Needs to Be Washed Twice a Week," *J Allergy
Clin Immunol*, 1999, 103: 581–585.

PAGE 133 **There are non-allergenic breeds of dog:** R. F. Lockey, "The Myth of
Hypoallergenic Dogs," *JACI*, October 2012, 130 (4): 910–911.

PAGE 133 **No relationship has yet been proved:** "Pet Allergies," acaai.org. http://
www.acaai.org/allergies/types/pet-allergy

PAGE 134 **Avian (bird) proteins:** "Goose Feathers," Thermo Scientific, 2012.
http://www.phadia.com/en/Products/Allergy-testing-products/ImmunoCAP
-Allergen-Information/Epidermals-and-Animal-Proteins/Allergens/Goose-
feathers/

PAGE 134 **But a recent study suggests:** A. L. Dryer et al, "Dust-Mite Allergen
Removal from Feathers by Commercial Processing," *Annals of Allergy, Asthma
& Immunology*, 2002, 88: 576–577.

J. F. Phillips and R. F. Lockey, "Exotic Pet Allergy," *J Allergy Clin
Immunol*, 2009, 123: 513–515.

PAGE 135 **There's evidence linking:** "Facts About Mold and Dampness," cdc.gov.
http://www.cdc.gov/mold/dampness_facts.htm

PAGE 135 **While mold is ever-present:** "Facts About Stachybotrys Chartarum
and Other Molds," National Center for Environmental Health, September 18,
2012. http://www.cdc.gov/mold/stachy.htm

PAGE 136 **Mold spores are found:** D. L. MacIntosh et al, "The Benefits of Whole-
House In-Duct Air Cleaning in Reducing Exposures to Fine Particulate
Matter of Outdoor Origin: A Modeling Analysis," *Journal of Exposure Science
and Environmental Epidemiology*, March–April 2010: 213–224.

PAGE 137 **The CDC's guidelines recommend mold prevention:** "Facts About
StachyBotrys Chartarum and Other Molds," CDC, September 18, 2012.
http://www.cdc.gov/mold/stachy.htm

PAGE 137 **Tips to Reduce Mold Exposure:** "Environmental Triggers of Asthma

Treatment, Management, and Prevention," from the Agency for Toxic Substances & Diseases Registry, an agency of the U.S. Department of Health and Human Services, November 28, 2014. http://www.atsdr.cdc.gov/csem/csem.asp?csem=32&po=9

Chapter 7: Skin Allergies

PAGE 142 **recent stressful events are often associated with the onset:** S. M. Dyke et al, "Effect of Stress on Basophil Function in Chronic Idiopathic Urticaria," *Clin Exp Allergy*, 2008, 38 (1): 86–92.

PAGE 142 **The mind-body connection:** "Recognizing the Mind-Skin Connection," Harvard Health Publications, November 2006. http://www.health.harvard.edu/newsletter_article/Recognizing_the_mind-skin_connection

PAGE 143 **Male skin tends to be oilier:** Diana Howard, "Is a Man's Skin Really Different?" The International Dermal Institute. http://www.dermalinstitute.com/us/library/17_article_Is_a_Man_s_Skin_Really_Different_.html

PAGE 144 **Roughly four in five children with eczema:** "Is Eczema in Kids Linked to Allergies and Asthma?" WebMD, 2016. http://www.webmd.com/skin-problems-and-treatments/eczema/child-eczema-16/allergies

J. A. Burgess et al, "Does Eczema Lead to Asthma?" *J Asthma*, June 2009, 46 (5): 429–436.

http://www.acaai.org/allergies/who-has-allergies/children-allergies/eczema

PAGE 145 **stress:** "Association of Stress with Symptoms of Atopic Dermatitis," *Acta Derm Venereol*, November 2010, 90 (6): 582–588.

PAGE 148 **yet the immune system:** A. Nosbaum, "Allergic and Irritant Contact Dermatitis," *Eur J Dermatol*, July–August 2009, 19 (4): 325–332.

PAGE 150 **a woman uses twelve types of personal care products daily:** "Exposures Add Up: Survey Results," ewg.org. http://www.ewg.org/skindeep/2004/06/15/exposures-add-up-survey-results/

PAGE 151 **It's estimated that 1 to 2 percent of the population:** Vanessa Ngan, "Fragrance Mix Allergy," DermNet New Zealand, 2002. http://www.dermnetnz.org/topics/fragrance-mix-allergy/

PAGE 151 **Fragrance is responsible:** Aria Vazirnia and Sharon E. Jacob, "Review ACDS' Allergen of the Year 2000–2015," November 2014. http://www.the-dermatologist.com/content/review-acds'-allergen-od-year-2000-2015

PAGE 154 **If you can't avoid contact with nickel:** "Nickel Allergy," Mayo Clinic, March 13, 2013. http://www.mayoclinic.org/diseases-conditions/nickel-allergy/basics/prevention/con-20027616

PAGE 155 **in Europe, limitations were placed on nickel:** "Nickel Release: New European Standards Released," Intertek, Sparkle,August 19, 2011, 596.

http://www.intertek.com/uploadedFiles/Intertek/Divisions/Consumer
_Goods/Media/PDFs/Sparkles/2011/sparkle596.pdf

PAGE 156 **Hives appear to afflict:** A paper presented at the World Allergy Congress in 2011 reported that women in their thirties were most likely to suffer from hives, World Allergy Organization XXII World Allergy Congress (WAC), Abstract 4072, presented December 7, 2011.

"Urticaria and Angiodema," World Allergy Organization, 2016. http://www.worldallergy.org/public/allergic_diseases_center/urticaria/urticaria.php

PAGE 160 **Approximately 2 to 5 percent:** Simone Laube, "Dermographism Urticaria," MedScape, March 29, 2016.
http://www.emedicine.medscape.com/article/1050294-overview

PAGE 160 **the link between less stress:** H-W. Chang et al, "Association Between Chronic Idiopathic Urticaria and Hypertension," *Ann Allergy Immunol*, 2016. https://www.univadis.com/viewarticle/hives-linked-to-hypertension-414959

PAGE 161 **Yoga: Although research says:** Erica Robinson, "Yoga Doesn't Help Asthma Sufferers Control Their Breathing Any Better Than Other Breathing Exercises," *Medical Daily*, June 8, 2014. http://www.medicaldaily.com/yoga-doesnt-help-asthma-sufferers-control-their-breathing-any-better-other-breathing-exercises

PAGE 161 **One study found that the benefits:** H. Cramer et al, "Yoga for Asthma: A Systematic Review and Meta-analysis," *Annals of Asthma, Allergy & Immunology*, 2014.

PAGE 161 **swimming has shown improvement:** Natasha Freutel, "Why Is Swimming Good for Asthma?" livestrong.com, December 11, 2015. http://www.livestrong.com/article/366684-why-is-swimming-good-for-asthma/

PAGE 161 **Biofeedback:** Richard J Martin, "Complementary, Alternative, and Integrative Therapies for Asthma," uptodate.com, February 2016. http://www.uptodate.com/contents/complementary-alternative-and-integrative-therapies-for-asthma

PAGE 161 **improved sleep quality is associated with better asthma control:** V. Cukic, "Sleep Disorders in Patients with Bronchial Asthma," Mater Sociomed, 2011, 23 (4): 235–237.

PAGE 162 **It takes only one-billionth of a gram:** Poison Ivy, Oak, & Sumac Information Center, 2016. http://www.poisonivy.aesir.com/view/fastfacts.html

PAGE 162 **oil can remain active for years:** "Poisonous Plants: Myths vs. Facts." http://www.goretexproducts.com/factsheets/2015/IvyX_myths2015.pdf

PAGE 167 **Many establishments, especially hospitals:** "Why Non-Latex?" Ansell, 2014. http://www.ansell.com/en-US/Campaigns/Non-Latex-Conversion/Why-Non-Latex/Why-Non-Latex.aspx

PAGE 167 **allergy to latex is considerably less common:** A. Heese et al, "Allergic and Irritant Reactions to Rubber Gloves in Medical Health Services: Spectrum, Diagnostic Approach, and Therapy," *J Am Acad Dermatol*, 1991, 25 (5, part 1): 831.

PAGE 167 **Latex paint does not contain:** "Does Latex Paint Contain Natural Rubber Latex?" American Latex Allergy Association, 2016. http://www.latex allergyresources.org/faqs/does-latex-paint-contain-natural-rubber-latex-nrl

PAGE 168 **Seminal plasma allergy:** Thomas H. Maugh, "New Research Confirms Semen Allergy in Some Men," *Medical Xpress*, January 9, 2011. http://www.phys.org/news/2011-01-semen-allergy-men.html#jCp; http://www.blogs.discovermagazine.com/seriouslyscience/2015/02/19/ can-allergic-semen/#.V9mLVSMrLgE

Chapter 8: Food Allergies

PAGE 170 **A ten-year longitudinal study:** L. Verrill, "Prevalence of Self-Reported Food Allergy in U.S. Adults: 2001, 2006, and 2010," *Allergy Asthma Proc*, November–December 2015, 36 (6): 458–467.

PAGE 170 **According to a survey cited by the Centers for Disease:** Kristen D. Jackson et al, "Trends in Allergic Conditions Among Children: United States, 1997–2011," Centers for Disease Control, May 2013. http://www.cdc.gov/nchs/ products/databriefs/db121.htm

PAGE 170 **Dr. Hugh Sampson, one of the country's:** Susan Dominus, "The Allergy Prison," *The New York Times*, June 10, 2001. http://www.nytimes .com/2001/06/10/magazine/the-allergy-prison.html

PAGE 170 **from 1997 to 2008 (as reported at three intervals):** Scott H. Sicherer et al, "U.S. Prevalence of Self-Reported Peanut, Tree Nut, and Sesame Allergy: 11-Year Follow-Up," *The Journal of Allergy and Clinical Immunology*, May 12, 2010.

PAGE 170 **six million US adults are allergic to shellfish or finned fish:** "Top 8: Fish and Shellfish," *AllergicChild*. http://www.home.allergicchild .com/top-8-fish/

PAGE 170 **In Europe, the last decade:** According to the European Academy of Allergy and Clinical Immunology, as referenced on "Facts and Statistics," at Food Allergy Research & Education (FARE). https://www.foodallergy.org/ facts-and-stats

PAGE 171 **Food-allergic kids are two to four times:** Amy M. Branum and Susan L. Lukacs, "Food Allergy Among U.S. Children: Trends in Prevalence and Hospitalizations," CDC, October 2008. http://www.cdc.gov/nchs/products/ databriefs/db10.htm

PAGE 171 **respiratory allergies:** Amy M. Branum and Susan L. Lukacs, "Food Allergy Among U.S. Children: Trends in Prevalence and Hospitalizations,"

CDC, October 2008. http://www.cdc.gov/nchs/products/databriefs/ db10.htm

PAGE 171 **these bacteria may shield us:** Robert Hotz, "Study Sees Link Between Allergies and the Infant Gut," *The Wall Street Journal*, October 10, 2016. http://www.wsj.com/articles/study-sees-link-between-allergies-and-the-infant -gut-1476122104

PAGE 171 **the Girl Scouts of America:** Susan Dominus, "The Allergy Prison," *The New York Times*, June 10, 2001. http://www.nytimes.com/2001/06/10/ magazine/the-allergy-prison.html

PAGE 171 **breathing in the steam of shellfish:** Daniel Ramirez, Jr., and Sami Bahna, "Food Hypersensitivity by Inhalation," *Clin Mol Allergy*, 2009, 7: 4.

PAGE 172 **Russian, Finnish and Estonian newborns:** Moises Velasquez-Manoff, "Educate Your Immune System," *The New York Times*, June 3, 2016. http:// www.nytimes.com/2016/06/05/opinion/sunday/educate-your-immune- system.html

PAGE 172 **As researchers Amy M. Branum and Susan L. Lukacs:** Amy M. Branum and Susan L. Lukacs, "Food Allergy Among U.S. Children: Trends in Prevalence and Hospitalizations," CDC, October 2008. http://www.cdc .gov/nchs/products/databriefs/db10.htm

PAGE 172 **We may be dealing with:** Robert Wood, quoted in "Milk and Egg Allergies Harder to Outgrow, Hopkins Study Shows," *Johns Hopkins Medicine*, December 11, 2007. http://www.hopkinsmedicine.org/news/media/ releases/milk_and_egg_allergies_harder_to_outgrow_hopkins_study_shows

PAGE 174 **a 2016 study showed that:** "Most Siblings of Food Allergic Kids Do Not Have Food Allergy," Ann & Robert H. Lurie Children's Hospital of Chicago, *ScienceDaily*, July 12, 2016. https://www.sciencedaily.com/ releases/2016/07/160712101224.htm

PAGE 174 **9 percent of kids tested positive for peanut allergies, yet just 1 percent developed:** "Siblings of Kids with Peanut Allergy May be Overprotected from Nuts," FairfieldCountyAllergy.com, January 1, 2015. http://www.fairfieldcountyallergy.com/siblings-kids-peanut-allergy-may -overprotected-nuts/

PAGE 175 **the majority of reactions were triggered:** David M. Flesicher et al, "Allergic Reactions to Foods in Preschool-Aged Children in a Prospective Observational Food Allergy Study," *Pediatrics*, July 2012, 130 (1). http://www .pediatrics.aappublications.org/content/130/1/e25

PAGE 176 **those at greatest risk of food-induced:** Allison J. Burbank et al, "Oral Immunotherapy for Food Allergy," *Immunol Allergy Clin North Am*, February 2016, 36 (1): 55–69.

PAGE 178 **[CHART]:** Modified from original, with appreciation to Judith C. Thalheimer, RD, LDN.

PAGE 180 **This condition is often found:** Y. Peng, "Polymorphism in East Asian Populations and Expansion of Rice Domestication in History," *BMC Evolutionary Biology*, 2010.

PAGE 179 **About 90 percent of food-allergic:** "Food Allergies: What You Need to Know," U.S. Food and Drug Administration, May 14, 2012. http://www .fda.gov/Food/ResourcesForYou/Consumers/ucm079311.htm

PAGE 181 **The incidence of children affected by food allergy:** "Food Allergy: A Practice Parameter," American College of Allergy, Asthma & Immunology, *Ann Allergy Asthma Immunol*, 2006, 96 (3, Suppl. 2): S1.

PAGE 181 **Among adults, the prevalence:** D. A. Moneret-Vautrin et al, "Adult Food Allergy," *Curr Allergy Asthma Rep*, 2005, 5 (1): 80.

PAGE 181 **How long it takes:** R. Gupta et al, "The Prevalence, Severity, and Distribution of Childhood Food Allergy in the United States," *Annals of Allergy, Asthma and Clinical Immunology*, July 2013.

PAGE 181 **On average, the younger the age:** R. Gupta et al, "The Prevalence, Severity, and Distribution of Childhood Food Allergy in the United States," *Annals of Allergy, Asthma and Clinical Immunology*, July 2013.

PAGE 181 **a food-allergic child has a 35 percent chance:** David A. Hill et al, "The Epidemiologic Characteristics of Healthcare Provider–Diagnosed Eczema, Asthma, Allergic Rhinitis, and Food Allergy in Children: A Retrospective Cohort Study," *BMC Pediatrics*, 2016, 16 (1).

PAGE 181 **On a happier note, children appear capable:** "Milk and Egg Allergies Harder to Outgrow, Hopkins Study Shows," *Johns Hopkins Medicine*, December 11, 2007. http://www.hopkinsmedicine.org/news/media/releases/ milk_and_egg_allergies_harder_to_outgrow_hopkins_study_shows

PAGE 182 **[from Milk: The #1 food allergy . . .]:** through the end of the list of the Big 8 food allergens (p. 179), the majority of listed, unboxed information is sourced from foodallergy.org. https://www.foodallergy.org/allergens, with their permission

PAGE 182 **The number one food allergy in infants:** Robert Wood, "Food Allergy in Children: Prevalence, Natural History, and Monitoring for Resolution," uptodate.com, July 12, 2016.

PAGE 182 **most children outgrow it:** Daniel More, "When Might My Child Outgrow His Milk Allergy?" December 10, 2015. https://www.verywell.com/ when-might-my-child-outgrow-his-milk-allergy-82843

PAGE 182 **The terms "nondairy":** "Food: Designation of Ingredients. In Food Labeling," Food and Drug Administration, 2004. Washington, D.C.: U.S. Government Printing Office via GPO Access. http://www.edocket.access .gpo.gov/cfr_2002/aprqtr/21cfr101.4.htm

Notes

PAGE 182 **It is required, however, that caseinates:** H. A. Sampson et al, "Safety of Casein Hydrolysate Formula in Children with Cow Milk Allergy," *J Pediatr*, April 1991, 118 (4, part 1): 520–525.

PAGE 185 **On very rare occasions:** J. M. Kelso, "Potential Food Allergens in Medications," *J Allergy Clin Immunol*, June 2014, 133 (6): 1509–1518.

PAGE 186 **By age sixteen, in one study:** "Egg Allergy," acaai.org. http://www .acaai.org/allergies/types/food-allergies/types-food-allergy/egg-allergy

PAGE 186 **Tolerance and frequent consumption of baked egg:** Robert Wood, "Food Allergy in Children: Prevalence, Natural History, and Monitoring for Resolution," uptodate.com, July 12, 2016.

PAGE 188 **Approximately 25 to 40 percent:** Jane Brody, "As Tree Allergies Rise, Trying to Determine a Cause," *The New York Times*, February 3, 2014 (correction at end of story). http://www.mobile.nytimes.com/blogs/ well/2014/02/03/as-peanut-allergies-rise-trying-to-determine-a-cause/

PAGE 190 **cleaning with antibacterial gel alone is not sufficient:** Tamara T. Perry et al, "Distribution of Peanut Allergen in the Environment," *Journal of Allergy and Clinical Immunology*, May 2004, 113 (5).

PAGE 190 **Only about 10 percent:** Miranda Hitti, "Study Shows About 9 Percent of Kids Eventually Outgrow Allergies to Tree Nuts," WebMD, November 9, 2005. http://www.webmd.com/allergies/news/20051109/nut-allergies-outgrown

PAGE 191 **Identifying problematic nuts:** T. L. Hostetler et al, "The Ability of Adults and Children to Visually Identify Peanuts and Tree Nuts," *Ann Allergy Asthma Immunol*, January 2012, 108 (1): 25–29.

PAGE 197 **in one study, more than half of kids:** "Wheat Allergy," acaai.org, 2014. http://www.acaai.org/allergies/types/food-allergies/types-food-allergy/ wheat-gluten-allergy

PAGE 202 **Soy allergy is often outgrown:** "Soy Allergy," American College of Allergy, Asthma & Immunology, 2014. http://www.acaai.org/allergies/types/ food-allergies/types-food-allergy/soy-allergy

PAGE 204 **Highly refined soybean oil:** "Soy Allergy," FARE, 2016. https://www .foodallergy.org/allergens/soy-allergy

PAGE 204 **allergic to sesame:** "Hypersensitivities to Sesame and Other Common Edible Seeds," *Allergy*, June 28, 2016. http://www.mdlinx.pdr.net/allergy- immunology/newsl-article.cfm/6727718/

PAGE 204 **would potentially add sesame to the list:** Cookson Beecher, "Sesame Gains Traction in Push for Food-Labeling Requirements," *Food Safety News*, November 30, 2015. http://www.foodsafetynews.com/2015/11/sesame-gaining- traction-in-congressional-push-for-food-labeling-requirements/#. V33PuCMrLmY

PAGE 209 **Anecdotally, it appears that the rate:** S. H. Sicherer, "Clinical Implications of Cross-Reactive Food Allergens," *J Allergy Clin Immunol,* December 2001, 108 (6): 881–890.

PAGE 211 **Kiwi allergy is also prevalent:** Jennifer Van Evra, "Serious Fruit Allergy: Kiwi," *AllergicLiving.* http://www.allergicliving.com/2010/09/01/serious-fruit-allergy-kiwi/

PAGE 221 **One conclusion reached: Families:** "Parents Give Variety of Reasons for Putting Off Food Challenges," *Kids With Food Allergies,* June 25, 2015. https://www.community.kidswithfoodallergies.org/blog/parents-give -researchers-reasons-why-they-avoid-oral-food-challenges-for-food-allergy

Chapter 9: Allergic and Non-Allergic Reactions to Drugs

PAGE 222 **The good news about true drug allergy:** "Medications and Drug Allergic Reactions," American Academy of Allergy, Asthma & Immunology. http://www.aaaai.org/conditions-and-treatments/library/at-a-glance/medications-and-drug-allergic-reactions

PAGE 223 **when a family of antibiotic drugs called fluoroquinolones:** On July 26, 2016, the U.S. Food and Drug Administration (FDA) approved changes to the labels of fluoroquinolone antibacterial drugs for systemic use.

PAGE 227 **Why do some people get drug allergy [whole passage]:** R. Mirakian et al, "BSACI Guidelines for the Management of Drug Allergy," *Clin Exp Allergy,* January 2009, 39 (1): 43–61.

PAGE 227 **A large study in the journal:** L. Zhou et al, "Drug Allergies Documented in Electronic Health Records of a Large Healthcare System," *Allergy,* September 2016, 71 (9): 1305–1313.

PAGE 229 **The number one cause of drug allergy:** "Medications and Drug Allergic Reactions," American Academy of Allergy, Asthma & Immunology. http://www.aaaai.org/conditions-and-treatments/library/at-a-glance/medications-and-drug-allergic-reactions

PAGE 229 **Serious reactions are common:** C. E. Lee et al, "The Incidence of Antimicrobial Allergies in Hospitalized Patients: Implication Regarding Prescribing Patterns and Emerging Bacterial Resistance," *Arch Intern Med,* 2000, 160: 2819; E. Macy et al, "Health Care Use and Serious Infection Prevalence Associated with Penicillin Allergy in Hospitalized Patients," *J Allergy Clin Immunolol,* 2014, 133: 790.

PAGE 230 **Some risk factors that may:** "Diseases and Conditions, Penicillin Allergy Risk Factors," Mayo Clinic. http://www.mayoclinic.org/diseases -conditions/penicillin-allergy/basics/risk-factors/con-200224205

PAGE 231 **Up to one-third of people:** Peter V. Dicpinigaitis, "Angiotensin-Converting Enzyme Inhibitor-Induced Cough," *Chest,* 2006, 129: 169S–173S.

PAGE 231 **Others may suffer a more serious reaction:** L. Zhou et al, "Drug Allergies Documented in Electronic Health Records of a Large Healthcare System," *Allergy*, September 2016, 71 (9): 1305–1313.

PAGE 233 **When certain fruits, vegetables:** "Patient Comments—Sun-Sensitive Drugs—Phototoxic Drugs," medicinenet. http://www.medicinenet.com/sun -sensitive_drugs_photosensitivity_to_drugs/patient-comments-2002.htm

PAGE 233 **One study found that the vast majority of patients:** S. R. Solensky and D. A. Khan, "Jt. Task Force on Practice Parameters: Drug Allergy: Summary Statement 7," *Annals of Allergy*, October 2010, 105.

PAGE 233 **allergy to local anesthetics during dental and/or other procedures:** J. C. Baluga, "Allergy to Local Anesthetic in Dentistry: Myth or Reality?" *Alerg Mex*, September–October 2003, 50 (5): 176–181.

S. J. Speca et al, "Allergy Reactions to Local Anesthetic Formulations," *Dental Clin North Am*, October 2010, 54 (4): 655–664.

PAGE 238 **If you are a woman:** P. Pradubpongsa et al, "Adverse Reactions to Iodinated Contrast Media: Prevalence, Risk Factors and Outcome: The Results of a 3-Year Period," *Asian Pac J Allergy Immunol*, December 2013, 31 (4): 299–306.

PAGE 238 **drug desensitization, has now been standardized:** Sloane et al, "Immunol— In Practice," *Journal of Allergy Clin*, May–June 2016, 4 (3): 497–504.

Chapter 10: Managing Allergy and Asthma, Today and Tomorrow

PAGE 244 **Think of when we blush:** "Recognizing the Mind–Skin Connection," Harvard Health Publications, November 2006. http://www.health.harvard .edu/newsletter_article/Recognizing_the_mind-skin_connection

PAGE 245 **They are exploring how stress:** P. Arck and R. Paus, "From the Brain–Skin Connection: The Neuroendocrine-Immune Misalliance of Stress and Itch," *Neuroimmunomodulation*, 2006, 13: 347–356.

PAGE 245 **Researchers are looking at how:** M. Jafferany et al, "Psychodermatology: Basic Concepts," *Act Derm Venerol*, 2016, Suppl. 217: 35–37. http://www.wjgnet.com/2218-6190/full/v2/i3/16.htm

R. A. Clay, "The Link Between Skin and Psychology," American Psychological Association, February 2015, 46 (2): 56.

PAGE 246 **the skin's permeability barrier, designed to keep out harmful:** Y. Chen and J. Lyga, "Brain–Skin Connection: Stress, Inflammation and Skin Aging," *Inflamm Allergy Drug Targets*, June 2014, 13 (3): 177–190;

"Mind–Body Connection May Extend to Skin," Harvard Health Publications. http://www.health.harvard.edu/press_releases/mind-body -connection;

A. L. Suarez et al, "Psychoneuroimmunology of Psychological Stress and

Atopic Dermatitis: Pathophysiologic and Therapeutic Updates," *Acta Derm Venereol,* January 2012, 92 (1): 7–15.

PAGE 247 **explore the non-medication strategies:** S. K. Agarwal and G. D. Marshall, Jr., "Stress Effects on Immunity and Its Application to Clinical Immunology," *Clinical and Experimental Allergy,* 2001, 31: 25–31. http://www .uth.tmc.edu/pathology/medic/immunology/Immuno/Agarwal-Marshall. stress.pdf

PAGE 247 **Consumer warnings have been issued:** Richard J. Martin, "Complementary, Alternative, and Integrative Therapies for Asthma," uptodate.com, February 2016. http://www.uptodate.com/contents/ complementary-alternative-and-integrative-therapies-for-asthma

PAGE 248 **antioxidants, vitamins A, C, D and E; soy isoflavones:** Richard J. Martin, "Complementary, Alternative, and Integrative Therapies for Asthma," uptodate.com, February 2016. http://www.uptodate.com/contents/ complementary-alternative-and-integrative-therapies-for-asthma

PAGE 249 **vitamin D levels appear to be:** Linda Searing, "Vitamin D May Help Cut Down Asthma Attacks," *Washington Post,* September 10, 2016. https:// www.washingtonpost.com/national/health-science/vitamin-d-may-help-cut -down-asthma-attacks/2016/09/09/9d612b20-7517-11e6-be4f-3f42f2e5a49e _story.html

A. R. Martineau et al, "Vitamin D for the Management of Asthma," *Cochrane Database of Systematic Reviews,* 2016, 8, article number CD011511.

PAGE 249 **data from Australia suggest:** E. M. Hollams, "Vitamin D Deficiency in Early Childhood Associated with Allergy, Asthma, and Eczema," *J Allergy Clin Immunol,* October 12, 2016. https://www.univadis.com/viewarticle/ vitamin-d-deficiency-in-early-childhood-associated-with-allergy-asthma-and -eczema-449534

PAGE 249 **concluded that greater vitamin D:** H. Feng et al, "In Utero Exposure to 25(OH) D and Risk of Childhood Asthma, Wheeze and Respiratory Tract Infections: A Meta-analysis of Birth Cohort Studies," *Journal of Allergy and Clinical Immunology,* September 16, 2016.

PAGE 250 **A German study among adults:** C. E. Ciaccio and Manika Girdhar, "The Effect of Maternal Omega 3 Fatty Acids Supplementation on Infant Allergy," *Ann Allergy Asthma and Immuno,* March 2014, 112 (3): 191–194.

PAGE 250 **omega-fatty acids:** "Omega 3 Fatty Acids May Reduce Children's Risk of Allergies," *Nutrition Facts,* July 26, 2012.

J. Miyata, "Role of Omega 3 Fatty Acids and Their Metabolites in Asthma and Allergic Disease," *Science Direct,* 2015.

Danielle Swanson et al, "Omega 3 Fatty Acids EP and DHA: Health Benefits Throughout Life," *Adv Nutr,* January 2012, 3 (1): 1–7.

PAGE 251 **Vitamin E, found in many edible nuts:** Ingrid Kolleck et al, "Vitamin E as an Antioxidant of the Lung," *American Journal of Respiratory and Critical Care Medicine*, December 15, 2002, 166 (Suppl. 1). http://www .atsjournals.org/doi/full/10.1164/rccm.2206019#.V98ZOCMrKX0

PAGE 251 **the mineral magnesium:** Richard J. Martin, "Complementary, Alternative, and Integrative Therapies for Asthma," uptodate.com, February 2016. http://www.uptodate.com/contents/complementary-alternative-and-integrative-therapies-for-asthma

PAGE 251 **Other studies point to the possible constructive impact that antioxidants:** C. Picado et al, "Dietary Micronutrients/Antioxidants and Their Relationship with Bronchial Asthma Severity," *Allergy European Journal of Allergy and Clinical Immunology*, January 2001.

S. O. Shaheen et al, "Dietary Antioxidants and Asthma in Adult Population–Based Case Study," *American Journal of Respiratory and Critical Care Medicine*, November 10, 2001, 164: 823–828.

J. A. Grieger et al, "Antioxidant-Rich Dietary Intervention for Improving Asthma Control in Pregnancy Complicated by Asthma: Study Protocol for a Randomized Controlled Study," *Trials*, April 4, 2014, 15: 108.

PAGE 251 **A study published in *Cell Reports*:** "Food Allergies Linked to Diet and Gut Microbiome," News Medical Life Sciences, June 21, 2016. http:// www.news-medical.net/news/20160621/Food-allergies-linked-to-diet-and -gut-microbiome.aspx

PAGE 251 **Caffeine is chemically similar:** Emma Welsh et al, "Caffeine for Asthma," Cochrane Database of Systematic Reviews, January 20, 2010.

PAGE 252 **Oranges: Asthmatic children who ate:** Francesco Forastiere et al, "Consumption of Fresh Fruit Rich in Vitamin C and Wheezing Symptoms in Children," *Thorax*, 2000, 55: 283–288. http://www.thorax.bmj.com/ content/55/4/283.full

PAGE 252 **A study from London's:** "Apples Protect the Lungs," BBC News, January 20, 2000. http://www.news.bbc.co.uk/2/hi/health/610068.stm

PAGE 252 **A Finnish study found:** S. M. Virtanen et al, "Early Introduction of Oats Associated with Decreased Risk of Persistent Asthma and Early Introduction of Fish with Decreased Risk of Allergic Rhinitis," *British Journal of Nutrition*, 2010, 103: 266–273.

PAGE 252 **A study found that for those suffering:** S. Masuda et al, "'Benifuuki' Green Tea Containing O-methylated Catechin Reduces Symptoms of Japanese Cedar Pollinosis: A Randomized, Double-Blind, Placebo-Controlled trial," *Allergol Int*, June 2014, 63 (2): 211–217. https://www.ncbi.nlm.nih.gov/ pubmed/24561771

PAGE 253 **development of atopy and asthma in kids:** F. M. Calatayud-Sáez et al, "Mediterranean Diet and Childhood Asthma," *Allergol Immunopathol*

(Madr), August 13, 2015. https://www.univadis.com/viewarticle/consumption -of-a-mediterranean-diet-and-childhood-asthma-297126

R. Barros et al, "Dietary Patterns and Asthma Prevalence, Incidence and Control," *Clinical and Experimental Allergy*, November 2015, 45 (11): 1673–1680.

M. A. Hendaus et al, "Allergic Diseases Among Children: Nutritional Prevention and Intervention," *Ther Clin Risk Man*, March 7, 2016, 12: 361–372.

PAGE 253 **The authors found that weight loss:** B. Folasade, "Weight Loss Interventions for Chronic Asthma," Editorial Group: Cochrane Airways Group, July 11, 2012.

PAGE 253 **The researchers' explanation for their findings?:** P. Ellwood et al, "Do Fast Foods Cause Asthma, Rhinoconjunctivitis and Eczema? Global Findings from the International Study of Asthma and Allergies in Childhood (ISAAC): Phase III," *Thorax*, 2012.

PAGE 254 **One or two studies provide hopeful results:** R. J. Bertelsen et al, "Probiotic Milk Consumption in Pregnancy and Infancy and Subsequent Childhood Allergic Diseases," *J Allergy Clin Immunol*, January 2014, 133 (1): 165–171.

John Gever, "Probiotics in Pregnancy Cuts Allergies in Tots," MedPage Today, February 25, 2013. http://www.medpagetoday.com/meetingcoverage/ aaaai/37521

PAGE 254 **another study found no benefit:** Wiley-Blackwell, "Probiotic Bacteria Don't Make Eczema Better, and May Have Side Effects, Study Shows," *ScienceDaily*, October 16, 2008. https://www.sciencedaily.com/ releases/2008/10/081007192433.htm

PAGE 254 **There's simply not enough evidence-based data:** "Probiotics for the Prevention of Allergy: A Systematic Review and Meta-analysis of Randomized Controlled Trials," meta-study of studies in Cochrane Central Register of Controlled Trials, MedLine and Embase, December 2014.

Meenu Singh, "Probiotic Effects in Allergic Disease," *Pediatric Allergy and Immunology*, March 2010, 21 (2, part 2): e368–e376.

PAGE 255 **For new parents, allergy awareness:** T. Polte et al, "Allergy Prevention Starts Before Conception: Maternofetal Transfer of Tolerance Protects Against the Development of Asthma," *J Allergy Clin Immunol*, November 2008, 122 (5): 1022–1030.e5.

PAGE 255 **In a large Danish study:** A. Sevelsted et al, "Cesarean Section and Chronic Immune Disorders," *Pediatrics*, January 2015, 135 (1): e92–e98.

PAGE 255 **possible association between C-section:** S. Thavagnanam et al, "A

Meta-analysis of the Association Between Caesarean Section and Childhood Asthma," *Clin Exp Allergy*, 2008, 38 (4): 629–633.e8.

H. Renz-Polster et al, "Caesarean Section Delivery and the Risk of Allergic Disorders in Childhood," *Clin Exp Allergy*, 2005, 35 (11): 1466–1472.

PAGE 256 **babies delivered by C-section:** E. Papathoma et al, "Cesarean Section Delivery and Development of Food Allergy and Atopic Dermatitis in Early Childhood," *Pediatr Allergy Immunol*, June 2016, 27 (4): 419–424.

PAGE 256 **The researchers observed:** C. Almqvist et al, "The Impact of Birth Mode of Delivery on Childhood Asthma and Allergic Diseases," *Clinical and Experimental Allergy*, September 2012, 42 (9): 1369–1376.

PAGE 256 **being born during pollen season:** G. A. Lockett, "Association of Season of Birth with DNA Methylation and Allergic Disease," *Allergy*, September 2016, 71 (9): 1314–1324.

PAGE 256 **exposure to a pet dog *before birth*:** Caroline Lodge et al, "Perinatal Cat and Dog Exposure and the Risk of Asthma and Allergy in the Urban Environment: A Systematic Review of Longitudinal Studies," *Clin Dev Immunol*, 2012: 176484.

PAGE 256 **Among various risk factors:** Richard deShazo and Stephen Kemp, "Allergic Rhinitis: Clinical Manifestations, Epidemiology, and Diagnosis," uptodate.com, October 22, 2014.

PAGE 256 **Interestingly, active smoking:** R. Kantor et al, "Association of Atopic Dermatitis with Smoking: A Systematic Review and Meta-analysis," *Journal of the American Academy of Dermatology*, August, 23, 2016.

PAGE 256 **use of paracetamol:** Nicholas Bakalar, "Tylenol During Pregnancy Tied to Asthma in Children," *The New York Times*, February 11, 2016. http://www.well.blogs.nytimes.com/2016/02/11/tylenol-during-pregnancy-tied-to-asthma-in-children/

PAGE 257 **strong association between receiving allergy:** "Allergy Shots During Pregnancy May Decrease Allergies in Children," *ScienceDaily*, November 2013. https://www.sciencedaily.com/releases/2013/11/131108090129.htm; http://www.acaai.org/news/allergy-shots-during-pregnancy-may-decrease-allergies-children

"Moms Who Got Allergy Shots While Pregnant May Help Prevent Allergies in Their Children," pregnancy.org (referencing ACAAI). http://www.pregnancy.org/content/moms-who-get-allergy-shots-while-pregnant-may-help-prevent-allergies-in-their-children

PAGE 257 **solid foods past 4 to 6 months:** Sherry Coleman Collins, "Can Food Allergies Be Prevented? Studies Show Introducing Risky Foods in Infancy

Lowers Incidence," *Today's Dietitian*, March 2013, 15 (3): 14. http://www
.todaysdietitian.com/newarchives/030413p14.shtml

PAGE 258 **The Israeli mothers:** G. Du Toit et al, "Early Consumption of Peanuts
in Infancy Is Associated with a Low Prevalence of Peanut Allergy," *J Allergy
Clin Immunol*, November 2008, 122 (5): 984–991.

PAGE 258 **A 2015 clinical trial:** George Du Toit et al, and Gideon Lack/
LEAP-On Study Team, "Effect of Avoidance on Peanut Allergy After
Early Peanut Consumption," *New England Journal of Medicine*, March 7,
2016.

PAGE 259 **A study of 533 pregnant women:** Jaclyn M. Coletta, "Omega-3 Fatty
Acids and Pregnancy," *Rev Obstet Gynecol*, Fall 2010, 3 (4): 163–171.

PAGE 259 **Some researchers have examined the effect:** A. Litonjua and S. Weiss,
"Risk Factors for Asthma," uptodate.com, September 30, 2011. http://www
.cursoenarm.net/uptodate/contents/mobipreview.
htm?27/40/28289?source=HISTORY#H32

P. Subbarao et al, "Asthma: Epidemiology, Etiology and Risk Factors,"
CMAJ, October 27, 2009, 181 (9): e181–e190.

PAGE 259 **beneficial impact on asthma:** F. M. Calatayud-Sáez at al,
"Mediterranean Diet and Childhood Asthma," *Allergol Immunopathol*
(Madr), August 13, 2015. https://www.univadis.com/viewarticle/consumption
-of-a-mediterranean-diet-and-childhood-asthma-297126

PAGE 259 **fish intake during pregnancy:** G. Q. Zhang et al, "Fish Intake
During Pregnancy or Infancy and Allergic Outcomes in Children: A
Systematic Review and Meta-analysis," *Pediatr Allergy Immunol*,
September 3, 2016.

PAGE 260 **more children need office visits to address:** M. Tollefson, A.
Bruckner, and Section on Dermatology, "Atopic Dermatitis: Skin-Directed
Management," *Pediatrics*, November 2014.

PAGE 260 **applying prescription emollient (moisturizer) to the skin of a
newborn:** K. Horimukai et al, "Application of Moisturizer to Neonates
Prevents Development of Atopic Dermatitis," *Journal of Allergy and Clinical
Immunology*, October2014, 134 (4): 824–830.e6.

E. L. Simpson et al, "A Pilot Study of Emollient Therapy for the Primary
Prevention of Atopic Dermatitis," *J Am Acad Dermatol*, October 2010, 63 (4):
587–593.

PAGE 261 **reducing the use of detergents:** E. L. Simpson et al, "Emollient
Enhancement of the Skin Barrier from Birth Offers Effective Atopic
Dermatitis Prevention," *JACI*, 2014, 134: 818–823.

PAGE 261 **physical training, including aerobic-type activities:** Kristin V.
Carson et al, "Physical Training for Asthma," Cochrane Airways Group,
September 30, 2013.

PAGE 261 **the possible benefit of swimming:** Natasha Freutel, "Why Is Swimming Good for Asthma?" livestrong.com, December 11, 2015. http://www.livestrong.com/article/366684-why-is-swimming-good-for-asthma/

PAGE 262 **Exercise-induced bronchoconstriction:** John M. Weiler et al, "Pathogenesis, Prevalence, Diagnosis, and Management of Exercise-Induced Bronchoconstriction: A Practice Parameter," *Annals of Allergy, Asthma & Immunology*, December 2010, 105.

PAGE 262 **One study reported:** M. E. Faulstich et al, "Psychophysiologcal analysis of atopic dermatitis," *J Psychosom res*, 1985, 29 (4): 415–417.

PAGE 262 **stress may play a role:** L. Rees, "An Aetiolgical Study of Chronic Urticaria and Angioedema," *J Psychosom Res*, 1957, 2 (3): 172–189.

PAGE 262 **Relaxation therapy and other related:** C. L. Shertzer et al, "Effects of Relaxation Therapy in Chronic Urticarial," *Arch Dermatol*, July 1987, 123 (7): 913–916.

PAGE 263 **One study of Buteyko:** Richard J. Martin, "Complementary, Alternative, and Integrative Therapies for Asthma," uptodate.com, February 2016. http://www.uptodate.com/contents/complementary-alternative-and -integrative-therapies-for-asthma

PAGE 264 **One study trained a cohort:** Richard J. Martin, "Complementary, Alternative, and Integrative Therapies for Asthma," uptodate.com, February 2016. http://www.uptodate.com/contents/complementary-alternative-and -integrative-therapies-for-asthma

PAGE 264 **For one month:** Richard J. Martin, "Complementary, Alternative, and Integrative Therapies for Asthma," uptodate.com, February 2016. http://www.uptodate.com/contents/complementary-alternative-and -integrative-therapies-for-asthma

PAGE 264 **In one test of eighty:** Richard J. Martin, "Complementary, Alternative, and Integrative Therapies for Asthma," uptodate.com, February 2016. http://www.uptodate.com/contents/complementary-alternative-and -integrative-therapies-for-asthma

PAGE 265 **significant differences in lung function:** M. A. Hondras et al, "Manual Therapy for Asthma," Cochrane Airways Group, April 2005.

PAGE 265 **acupuncture was associated with a reduction:** B. Brinkhaus, "Acupuncture and Chinese Herbal Medicine in the Treatment of Patients with Seasonal Allergic Rhinitis: A Randomized-Controlled Clinical Trial," *Pediatrics*, December 2010, 126 (6).

B. Brinkhaus et al, "Acupuncture in Patients with Seasonal Allergic Rhinitis: A Randomized Trial," *Ann Intern Med*, February 2013, 158 (4): 225–234.

PAGE 266 **This is an often helpful approach:** B. Engin et al, "Treatment of Chronic Urticaria with Narrowband Ultraviolet B Phototherapy: A Randomized Controlled Trial," *Acta Derm Venereol*, 2008, 88: 247–251.

Notes

PAGE 266 **a recent Finnish study reached the same conclusion:** E. Lee et al, "UVB Phototherapy and Skin Cancer Risk: A Review of the Literature," *Pub Med. Int Dermatology Journal*, May 2005, 44 (5): 355–360.

PAGE 267 **sleep disturbances are associated:** Z. Li et al,"Longitudinal Associations Among Asthma Control, Sleep Problems, and Health-Related Quality of Life in Children with Asthma," *Sleep Med*, 2016, 20: 41–50. https://www.univadis.com/viewarticle/better-sleep-may-improve-childhood -asthma-418373;

V. Cukic et al, "Sleep Disorders in Patients with Asthma," *Mater Sociomed*, 2011, 23 (4): 235–237.

PAGE 268 **Several studies have found:** G. B. Panjo et al, "Asthmatic Children Mono Sensitized to House Dust Mite by Specific Immunotherapy: A Six-Year Follow-Up Study," *Clinical and Experimental Allergy*, September 2001, 31 (9): 1392–1397;

J. Schmitt et al, "Allergy Immunotherapy for Allergic Rhinitis Effectively Prevents Asthma: Results from a Large Retrospective Cohort Study," December 2015, 136 (6): 1511–1516.

PAGE 268 **Immunotherapy has been shown to reduce asthma symptoms:** L. Cox et al, "Allergen Immunotherapy: A Practice Parameter, Third Update," *J Allergy Clin Immunol*, January 2001, 127 (1): S1–S55;

J. Corren, "The Connection Between Allergic rhinitis and bronchial asthma," *Curr Opin Pulm Med*, 2007, 13 (1): 13;

L. Jacobsen et al, "Specific Immunotherapy Has Long-Term Preventive Effect of Seasonal and Perennial Asthma: 10-Year Follow-Up on the PAT Study," *Allergy*, 2007, 62 (8): 943;

L. Jacobsen et al, "How Strong Is the Evidence That Immunotherapy in Children Prevents the Progression of Allergy and Asthma?" *Curr Opin Allergy Clin Immunol*, 2007, 7 (6): 556.

PAGE 268 **Allergy injection immunotherapy:** "SLIT Treatment (Allergy Tablets) for Allergic Rhinitis Nothing to Sneeze About," American Academy of Allergy, Asthma & Immunology. http://www.aaaai.org/conditions-and -treatments/library/allergy-library/sublingual-immunotherapy-for-allergic -rhinitis

PAGE 269 **patients with asthma and house dust mite:** J. C. Virchow, "Efficacy of a House Dust Mite Sublingual Allergen Immunotherapy Tablet in Adults With Allergic Asthma: A Randomized Clinical Trial," *JAMA*, April 26, 2016, 315 (16): 1715–1725.

PAGE 269 **A recent clinical trial looked at the benefit of giving very small, controlled amounts of egg to egg-allergic children:** Jean-Christoph Caubet and Julie Wang, "Current Understanding of Egg Allergy," *Pediatric Clinics of North America*, April 1, 2011, 58 (2): 427–433.

PAGE 271 **The Veta is a smart case:** "Latest Mobile Tech Devices Look to
Improve Food Allergy, Asthma Safety," *Kids with Food Allergies*, January 30,
2015. http://www.community.kidswithfoodallergies.org/blog/latest-mobile
-tech-devices-look-to-improve-food-allergy-asthma-safety-1

PAGE 272 **researchers at MIT:** Anne Trafton, "Asthma Linked to DNA
Damage," *MIT News*, May 2, 2016. http://www.news.mit.edu/2016/asthma
-linked-dna-damage-0502

Index

■

Page numbers in **bold** indicate tables or charts; those in *italics* indicate figures; those followed by "n" indicate notes.

Index

nasal allergy, 56–58
nasal breathing exercises, 263
nasal decongestants, 57, 59, 61, 63, 82, 110
nasal endoscopy, 64, 67
nasal irrigation, 59–61, 64, 65
nasal priming, 84
nasal steroids, 54, 57, 61, 62, 63, 67, 84, 110, 273
    See also steroids
National Allergy Bureau (NAB), 90, 91, 108
National Center for Complementary and Integrative Health, 60–61
National Institute for Occupational Safety and Health (NIOSH), 95, 95n
National Institutes of Health, 45–46
National University of Singapore, 272
Natural Resources Defense Council, 7
neomycin, 150, 227
neti pots, 60, 61, 65, 66
neuroimmunology, 160, 243–44, 244–45
new allergy solution, ix–x, 14–18, 22, 37–41, 42, 43, 49–50
    See also allergies, the; asthma; children; defining the terms, diagnosing the problem; immune system; managing allergy and asthma; medications for allergies; prevention
New England Journal of Medicine, 258
new ways. *See* managing allergy and asthma
new weather map/seasons, 6, 162–63
nickel and other metals, 7, 34, 139, 143, 148, 150, 154–55, 247
nitrates/nitrites, 218
non-allergic drug reactions, 222, 223–24, 233–34, 273
non-allergic rhinitis, 53, 54, 58–61, 62, 63
nonceliac gluten sensitivity, 15, 47, 173, **178,** 198, 199, 200, 215
"nondairy" label, 182
non-medication, skin allergies, 142
nonsteroidal anti-inflammatory drugs (NSAIDs), 10, 35, 69, 157, 210, 222, 223, 228, 231, 232, 237
non-steroidal spray (cromolyn), 63
North American Contact Dermatitis Group, 155
nose and sinuses. *See* basic allergies

oak moss, 151
obesity, 9, 12, 46, 253

observations, identifying allergies, 38
occupational exposure, 9, 37, 46, 69, 70, **140,** 148, 153
ocular drops, 64, 81, 110
odd triggers, 9
Ogren, Tom, 5, 99
Ogren Plant Allergy Scale (OPALS), 92, *99,* 99–100
Ohio State University, 115
Old Friends Hypothesis, 31
olopatadine (Pantanol, Pazeo), 77
omega-fatty acids, 250
onset of drug reaction, 224, 225
opiates, 157, 231
oral allergy syndrome (OAS) and cross-reactivity, 100–101, 167, 171, 173, 176, 208–14, *213–14,* 219–20
oral contact dermatitis, 211
oral decongestants, 61, 63, 110, 225
oral food challenge (OFC), **178,** 181, 220–21
oral leukotriene receptor blocker (montelukast), 63
oranges, 252
outdoor and seasonal allergies, 33, 83–111
    See also specific allergies
outgrowing food allergy, 181–82
overcleaning (hygiene hypothesis), 7n, 7–8, 30, 31–36
overmedication (symptom management), 7, 17, 273
overtesting for food allergies, 174
over-the-counter (OTC) medications, 61, 65, 86, 104, 106, 110, 118, 124, 139, 146, 147, 149, 150, 185, 215, 222, 225, 235, 237
ozone, 6, 20, 85, 89, 164

paper wasps, 103
parabens, 150, 217
paraphenylenediamine (PPD), 34, 152–54
parasites, 30–31, 177
patch test, 39, 81, 147, 149, 151–52, 153–54, 155–56, 165, 181, 227, 229, 269
peaches, 100, 173, 210, 211, *213*
peanuts, peanut allergy
    basic allergies, 53
    defining and diagnosing, 29, 30, 34
    food allergies, 170, 171, 173, 174, 176, 179, 180, 181, 188–90, 191, 202, 210, 212, 214, 219, 220

Index

Index